THE
AIDS PANDEMIC

**Recent Titles in
Contributions in Medical Studies**

THE AIDS PANDEMIC

Social Perspectives

Yole G. Sills

Contributions in Medical Studies, Number 38

GREENWOOD PRESS
Westport, Connecticut • London

Library of Congress Cataloging-in-Publication Data

Sills, Yole G.
  The AIDS pandemic : social perspectives / Yole G. Sills.
    p. cm.—(Contributions in medical studies, ISSN 0886-8220 ;
  no. 38)
  Includes bibliographical references and index.
  ISBN 0-313-28606-X (alk. paper)
  1. AIDS (Disease)—Social aspects. I. Title. II. Series.
  RA644.A25S55 1994
   362.1'969792—dc20   93-25064

British Library Cataloguing in Publication Data is available.

Library of Congress Catalog Card Number: 93-25064
ISBN: 0-313-28606-X
ISSN: 0886-8220

First published in 1994

Greenwood Press, 88 Post Road West, Westport, CT 06881
An imprint of Greenwood Publishing Group, Inc.

Printed in the United States of America

The paper used in this book complies with the
Permanent Paper Standard issued by the National
Information Standards Organization (Z39.48-1984).

10 9 8 7 6 5 4 3 2 1

Contents

Preface

This book seeks to give the general reader an overview of the social, economic, and political impact that AIDS is having throughout the world. The sudden appearance and rapid spread of AIDS has spawned a sometimes bewildering spate of articles, books, and press commentaries that, taken together, provide an enormous amount of information about this disease and its social impact. For the nonspecialist seeking orientation and understanding, the problem is where to begin. This book offers a summary of recent writings about AIDS and a framework for thinking about and assessing the AIDS pandemic. For the specialist in one aspect of AIDS, the book provides an overview of its broader social aspects. For all readers, it introduces a rich array of research reports from many fields that documents the social origins and impacts of AIDS.

The sources used for this summary cover a wide range of fields, principally anthropology, demography, economics, epidemiology, history, medicine, political science, public health, social psychology, and sociology. This range is required because AIDS is at once a scientific, a medical, and a social problem. The problems created by AIDS require that we understand the methods and knowledge of all these disciplines in order to grasp their full meaning and to grope for solutions. AIDS is a social event of great magnitude, not simply a series of individual tragedies or a major chapter in the history of disease.

The magnitude of AIDS as a social event is a major concern of this book. Here it can only be noted that quite apart from the problems inherent in any disease of epidemic proportions is the social context in which it is occurring. A major focus of the book is the international context, that is, the AIDS pandemic.

Attention is also given to the social context in which the epidemic in the United States is taking place—specifically, a time of increased sensitivity to civil rights, and particularly to the civil rights of minorities; a social climate of both increased tolerance for unconventional life-styles and widespread sexual permissiveness; and a period of intense concern with ethical considerations relating to the care of the sick. The AIDS crisis has focused attention on major fissures in democratic societies. It has created policy conflicts, ethical dilemmas, and contradictions on various levels of government—from cities and towns to nations and the United Nations—concerning responsibility for the prevention of illness and for the care of the sick and others who have fallen by the wayside.

This overview does not include the specialized literature on the biology of AIDS. Researchers, immunologists, and clinicians can, of course, obtain current information from their professional journals; for the general reader, excellent reviews of knowledge about AIDS and of the prospects for a cure and a vaccine are periodically published in such journals as *Science* and *Scientific American*, as well as in the news weeklies. Also omitted for the most part is the literature that deals with the psychological trauma facing AIDS patients and their families and friends, as they contemplate and face a premature and painful death, as well as the literature aimed at the medical, nursing, and social work professionals who attend to AIDS patients and their families. Inclusion of these topics would require a separate volume.

The book originated as a project of the Center for Intercultural Education at Ramapo College of New Jersey, and I am deeply indebted to its director, John Robert Cassidy, for his encouragement and support. With his imaginative leadership of interdisciplinary studies, Bob Cassidy has enriched the life of Ramapo College from its founding. Robert Scott, president of Ramapo College, has supported the project since its beginning.

Norman N. Miller of Dartmouth College, the founder and editor of the journal *AIDS & Society*, first introduced me to the problem of AIDS in Africa through his pioneering book of that title (co-edited with Richard C. Rockwell), and has been a source of advice and encouragement ever since.

During the years 1978 through 1989, when I served as director of interdisciplinary studies at Ramapo, the college sponsored a number of seminars, workshops, television programs, and academic courses on the relationship of science and technology to society. The programs devoted to AIDS constituted the direct impetus for the preparation of the book.

Norma Yueh, director of the Ramapo College Library, and members of her staff, provided much-needed assistance in searching the voluminous literature on AIDS, as did the librarians of the Columbia School of Public Health and the outstanding public libraries of Darien and Greenwich, Connecticut. My own knowledge of the research literature was considerably enhanced by my participation in the Fourth International Conference on AIDS, held in Stockholm in June 1989. Ramapo College supported my travel to Stockholm, and I am very thankful for this assistance.

Among the many AIDS researchers whose writings are summarized in this book, I am particularly indebted to these scholars for personal consultations: Francis Paine Conant, Hunter College, City University of New York; Daniel M. Fox, Milbank Memorial Fund; Rosa Haritos, Columbia University; Carol Levine, Citizens Commission on AIDS for New York and Northern New Jersey; Norman N. Miller, Dartmouth College and *AIDS & Society*; Priscilla Reining, American Association for the Advancement of Science; Sebastian Rinken, European University Institute, Florence; Richard C. Rockwell, University of Michigan; and David E. Wilder, School of Public Health, Columbia University. The first draft of the manuscript was read by John Robert Cassidy; Edward Saiff, director of Ramapo's School of Theoretical and Applied Science; David L. Sills; and Elaine Winshell, professor of biology at Ramapo College. All provided many helpful comments.

David L. Sills, editor of the *International Encyclopedia of the Social Sciences*, provided skillful and efficient editorial and bibliographical services; Richard Katzman of Katzman Associates and C. P. Wolf of the Social Impact Assessment Center served willingly as volunteer computer consultants. It is a pleasure to record that I am eternally indebted to them all.

THE
AIDS PANDEMIC

1

Introduction:
A Profile of the
Pandemic

In the 1990s the AIDS pandemic is in its second decade and is continuing unabatedly; no country has been able to stop its growth. Moreover, it is spreading to hitherto untouched regions. It is an ongoing, evolving phenomenon that has for the most part inspired apocalyptic appraisals and doomsday scenarios concerning its impact. Using any standard of measure—deaths, the number of people infected with lingering and debilitating illness, the growth in the orphaned population, the decimation of the labor force, social and economic costs—AIDS may not be another Black Death, but it is a major global catastrophe nonetheless. Moreover, there is general agreement among scientists and public health officials that AIDS is here to stay, for a long time to come. Perhaps even more than malnutrition, whose cure is well known, AIDS is the disease that seems destined to characterize the end of the twentieth century and much of the twenty-first.

AIDS was not authoritatively identified as a new disease until 1981. Soon thereafter, the appearance of small clustered outbreaks of cases in various regions of the world—in Africa, the Caribbean, Europe, Latin America, and the United States—defined it as a true pandemic.

Awareness of the magnitude of this event—of the fact that AIDS had spread this rapidly and this widely—came only gradually. Knowledge concerning the number of diagnosed cases, the number of people who had succumbed, and the growing number who were infected with the lethal human immunodeficiency virus (HIV), but did not yet have AIDS, became available in slow stages. (In contrast, knowledge of the nature of the causative agent of the disease and of its pathology was acquired quite rapidly.) By the middle of the 1980s, and then increasingly as 1990 approached, the full dimensions of the worldwide catastrophe and its potential were revealed.

⌐ Early in the second AIDS decade, there is ample evidence that the pandemic has spread to six continents and to many islands as well. Furthermore, it has become painfully evident that it is intensifying in all affected areas. What is also increasingly apparent is the rapidly changing profile of the pandemic. According to a massive report on the pandemic, *AIDS in the World*, edited by Jonathan Mann and his colleagues at the Harvard AIDS Institute, the pandemic is "dynamic, unstable, and volatile" (1992:15–19).[1] In effect, it consists of many different epidemics with different time scales. As it matures, it becomes more complex, and it is now composed of thousands of smaller complicated epidemics. Moreover, the researchers see signs that the pandemic may be "out of control," that its course through many societies has yet to be influenced in any substantial way, and that its major impact is yet to come.

The scale of the pandemic

Precise estimates of the severity of the pandemic and projections of its future course are still largely matters of conjecture. The difficulties inherent in making precise estimates are described in a 1992 report of the U.S. Department of State, *The Global AIDS Disaster: Implications for the 1990s,* as follows:

> No country has an accurate count of the number of people infected by the Human Immunodeficiency Virus. Much of the testing to date comprises small samples of high-risk groups, such as prostitutes and drug addicts, and is therefore unrepresentative of entire populations. Within countries, infection rates vary widely from region to region, further complicating the problem of generalizing from a small sample. Counting the number of Acquired Immune Deficiency Syndrome cases

---

[1] Jonathan Mann, a public health physician, resigned in March 1989 from his position as director of the Global Programme on AIDS of the World Health Organization (WHO) to become director of the International AIDS Center at Harvard University's AIDS Institute. Michael Merson succeeded him at the WHO. Mann's co-editors in the preparation of *AIDS in the World* were Daniel J. M. Tarantola, a public health specialist formerly with WHO, and Thomas W. Netter, a communications consultant at the Harvard School of Public Health.

and AIDS-related deaths is also difficult, particularly since health care systems in many countries lack the required diagnostic ability. Moreover, some governments suppress what information they have. Further improvements in data collection will probably reveal a crisis of even greater magnitude than is portrayed in this study (U.S. Department of State 1992:vi).

Tentative as the data are, the emerging profile and its long-term implications become clearer as reports of the number of cases of AIDS and estimates of the number of individuals who are infected with HIV are periodically revised.

A voluminous and burgeoning literature on the pandemic documents the discrepancies in estimates of the number of individuals who have become ill with AIDS, the number who have died, and the larger number who have been infected with HIV but are still free of symptoms. These discrepancies are the result of a complex of factors, rooted in the elusive, insidious, and confusing nature of AIDS, its long incubation period, its political sensitivity, and its social dilemmas. Compounding these factors is the scarcity of resources and organizational mechanisms for tracking the spread of the disease in much of the world.

The frustration resulting from these uncertainties has been graphically described by Marsha Goldsmith:

> Increasing incidence and prevalence worldwide is the loud and clear message regarding the spread of acquired human immunodeficiency syndrome (AIDS), but when one tries to pin down just what is happening where, the numbers are found to be soft and the story often confused.
>
> While information issued by the World Health Organization (WHO) and gathered at recent meetings in this country and abroad contributes to understanding the current sway of immunodeficiency virus (HIV), it must be realized that seldom has so much data been presented by so many in so qualified a manner. Even when exact figures are given, as they often are, it is tacitly understood that what one is really hearing is a best guess based on the limited facts available (Goldsmith 1988:46).

Much the same situation prevails in the 1990s in the developing world, although in the last few years some improvements in the reporting of AIDS cases have been made.

James Chin, chief of the Surveillance, Forecasting, and Impact Assessment Division of the WHO Global Programme on AIDS, has repeatedly warned that case-reporting statistics are highly distorted. Reported interregional variations in AIDS incidence are in part the result of incomplete and delayed data. The completeness of reporting is said to vary from 90 percent for some industrialized countries to less than 10 percent for some developing countries. As pointed out by Chin (quoted in *Science*, Research News, April 19, 1991), WHO officials know that some developing countries report only 5 to 10 percent of the actual number of cases. Moreover, according to Chin, cases that were diagnosed in the early 1980s continued to be reported as new cases as late as 1989. As Jonathan Mann (1988a:16) has explained, "we can only know what individual countries tell us. There is no country in the world today, including, the United States, France, Sweden, and the United Kingdom, with a really accurate estimate." In the United States, which has a sophisticated surveillance network, almost 18 percent of all AIDS cases are unreported—according to the Centers for Disease Control and Prevention (CDC) in Atlanta, Georgia, the U.S. government agency that conducts epidemiological research for the Department of Health and Human Services.[2]

In an assessment of the CDC system of reporting AIDS cases, the National Research Council's Committee on AIDS Research and the Behavioral, Social, and Statistical Sciences (Turner et al. 1989:32–33) highlighted two problems: (1) in the United States only 85 to 90 percent of all new cases of AIDS are reported within one year of diagnosis; and (2) the reliability and validity with which the mode of transmission is established in each case have not been evaluated.

Problems in counting cases

While at the WHO, Mann and his colleagues (1988:82) identified three basic reasons for confusion over the number of AIDS cases in Africa and elsewhere in the developing world: "underrecognition, underdiagnosis and underreporting." The fundamental causes of all these uncertainties are rooted in the very nature of AIDS, as well as, ultimately, in the nature of the social

---

[2] The periodic *HIV/AIDS Surveillance* reports of the CDC routinely include, under Technical Notes, statements that the data are provisional and that reporting delays vary widely and have been as long as several years in some cases.

contexts in which it occurs.

AIDS is a fatal affliction, with a complicated symptomology. The CDC, whose pioneering studies have served to define the nature of AIDS throughout the world, refers to it on the cover of *HIV/AIDS Surveillance* as "a specific group of diseases or conditions which are indicative of severe immunosuppression related to infection with the human immunodeficiency virus (HIV)." Although it was originally seen as having a random collection of symptoms that were characterized as a syndrome, AIDS eventually turned out to be a disease with a single cause—the HIV.[3]

The definitive diagnosis of AIDS is based on the laboratory analysis of an individual's blood. But in many developing countries, where sophisticated laboratory testing facilities are not available or are too expensive to use, diagnosis has depended on the analysis of clinical symptoms using definitions devised by the WHO. Discrepancies have arisen between the CDC and the WHO definitions, which have further complicated determining the accuracy of case reports from African countries. Diagnosis based on the recognition of clinical symptoms by physicians is complicated by the fact that the HIV attacks and eventually destroys the immune system in slow stages, rendering patients vulnerable to a spectrum of opportunistic infections. These infections, which may vary by geographic area, are caused by organisms that are prevalent locally. The classic first symptoms of AIDS, weight loss and diarrhea, are recognized the world over. (In sub-Saharan Africa, AIDS is called "slim disease.") These symptoms are often untreated as such in some developing countries. Since in Africa and in other tropical areas such as the Caribbean, diarrhea is a commonly reported cause of death, thousands of cases of AIDS deaths may be misdiagnosed. In Africa, which has been hard hit by the epidemic, the difficulty of diagnosing AIDS infection clinically is considered one of the main problems in determining its prevalence. AIDS symptoms, moreover, can mimic other diseases. Even in the United States, according to James Goedert of the National Cancer Institute, AIDS can initially resemble chicken pox, measles, and other diseases that are more severe in adults than in children (quoted in Packard & Epstein 1992:367).

Compounding the difficulties inherent in the nature of AIDS in the developing world are the inadequate training received by

---

[3] For an account of the investigation that led to the discovery of the AIDS virus, see Robert C. Gallo's *Virus Hunters* (1991). At the 1992 AIDS conference in Amsterdam, reports were given of a few AIDS patients who were said not to have the HIV virus.

many doctors, the lack of trained laboratory technicians, and the lack of transportation for delivering blood samples to laboratories.

The separate problem of the underreporting of cases to national health authorities is largely a function of the inadequacies of all medical services in many countries. African countries in particular are plagued by a shortage of physicians: there is an average of one physician for every 20,000 people in sub-Saharan Africa, compared to one for every 800 in the United States. Demographers also blame the lack of surveillance systems in Africa for the underreporting of AIDS cases. Furthermore, the number of cases reported may not reflect the actual number of diagnosed cases because of internal delays in sending the data to national health authorities as well as to WHO.

Another cause of underreporting is that in regions where tuberculosis is endemic and many people die from it, the cause of death may be listed as TB, rather than AIDS, which in fact may be the prime cause. Chin, noting how TB rates have been "shooting up," remarks that "you can't kill a person twice." The reporting dilemma is whether to describe a death as "a TB death or an HIV death with tuberculosis or a TB death with HIV." "My recommendation," Chin adds playfully, "is we keep double books" (quoted in *Science*, Research News, April 19, 1991:373). Still another deterrent to accurate reporting, particularly on the African continent, is rooted in cultural norms. Dieter Koch-Weser (1988:xi) stresses that AIDS is a disease that bears "a dreadful social and, in the eyes of many, even moral stigma." Accordingly, it is underreported.

Because of all these difficulties, the official quarterly reports of the Surveillance, Forecasting, and Impact Assessment Division of the Global Programme on AIDS are universally recognized as conveying only a partial picture of the scale of the pandemic. However, they do provide crucial information concerning the relative size of epidemics occurring in different regions of the world—if we assume that the amount of underreporting is relatively universal. In January 1993, WHO reported that at the end of 1992 there had been 600,000 reported cases of AIDS worldwide, but that the real total was probably four times as high (*New York Times*, January 16, 1993:3). Jonathan Mann et al. (1992:2) estimate that 2.7 million people in the world have thus far had AIDS, of whom more than 90 per cent have died.

HIV infection: The invisible pandemic

Estimates of the severity of the pandemic distinguish between the number of individuals who have developed symptoms—and have accordingly been diagnosed as having AIDS—and the number of individuals who are infected with HIV but who don't yet have symptoms. In effect, the most observable aspects of the epidemic represent only a fraction of the total picture. As Mann and his colleagues point out in *AIDS in the World*, the major impact of the pandemic is yet to come because of the time that elapses between an individual's becoming infected and the onset of AIDS.

Because of this unique characteristic of AIDS, there are two pandemics: one of clinically diagnosed cases of sick people succumbing to the ravages of the fatal disease of AIDS and another, invisible pandemic consisting of people who are not yet sick but are contaminated by the HIV and can transmit it to others. Most are slated eventually to succumb to AIDS and die. The scope of both pandemics constantly changes as new data become available.

Estimates of the number and the characteristics of people who have become infected but are not sick are crucial. These estimates provide information about what kinds of people are most at risk of falling victim to AIDS; they are a further indication of the growth of an epidemic within a particular region; and ultimately they reveal the magnitude of the entire pandemic. As a number of epidemiologists put it, they are a window on the future.

Because HIV infection is clinically invisible, information on its spread must be obtained through serological surveys that analyze blood tests of representative samples of a population. WHO encourages standardized serological surveillance of HIV as the most reliable means of assessment—and of forecasting infection rates in developing countries. In the United States, the Centers for Disease Control collaborate with municipal and state departments of health as well as with a variety of other agencies, including blood banks, in order to obtain this information. But here again researchers encounter the same problem of the paucity of data in developing countries as they encounter in obtaining adequate reports of diagnosed cases. In Africa, for example, there has been no large-scale survey of seroprevalence based on nationally representative samples of the population: estimates of the infection rate are based on extrapolations from many small-scale surveys. These surveys, which are growing in number, are derived from blood tests of special target groups chosen chiefly for their availability. They include prostitutes, blood donors, women visiting clinics, and hospital patients. Although indicative, these data are not representative of the population at large and are thus flawed to the same extent as the data on case reporting.

Linda Valleroy (1988:49) has stressed a basic limitation of HIV seroprevalence studies, namely, that "it is not clear what the correspondence is, in a population between the number of people with AIDS and the number infected with HIV." Numerous assumptions are made to compensate for this limitation. "A common assumption is that for every person who has AIDS there are 100 people who are infected with the virus but show no symptoms," Valleroy reports. This assumption is the basis for the so-called "tip of the iceberg" or "tip of the pyramid" metaphors used to describe the epidemic. The 100 to 1 assumption has little scientific basis, given the facts that AIDS cases are underreported. Valleroy notes that "no country has yet completed a national seroprevalence study based on a representative sample."

No matter how flawed they are, existing seroprevalence surveys do add to our cumulative knowledge about epidemiological patterns of infection and provide a basis for rough estimates of the number of people infected with the AIDS virus in the developing world. Peter Piot and his colleagues (1988a) at the Institute of Tropical Medicine in Antwerp maintain that—although many of the early studies were flawed because of problems associated with the particular blood test used (the so-called ELISA test[4])—most of these problems have been resolved and the data from serologic surveys have provided a fairly reliable picture of the spread of HIV infection throughout the world.

In the United States, estimates of the prevalence of HIV infection in the population are necessarily derived from the screening of such available groups as military recruits, pregnant women, and volunteer blood donors, and by making extrapolations from these counts. These data have obvious limitations: an accurate estimate would require obtaining blood samples from a representative sample of the entire population.

In spite of all these limitations on precision, the two major compilers of statistics on HIV infection are in close agreement on the number to be reported. The Harvard AIDS Institute estimates that

---

[4] ELISA is an acronym for enzyme-linked immunosorbent assay. A simpler, more economical method of serum analysis has been devised for use in developing countries and was tested in Kenya and Thailand in 1990–91. Suitable for use in rural hospitals, blood banks, and transfusion centers, it takes less than 20 minutes to complete and costs about 25 cents per sample. The U.S. government and the Rockefeller Foundation funded its development.

as of January 1, 1992, there were 12.9 million cases of HIV infection in the world (Mann et al. 1992:27), while in June 1993, the WHO announced that there were then some 14 million cases (*New York Times*, June 6, 1993:20).

Predicting the future of the pandemic

From the beginning of the pandemic speculations have been rife concerning the number of people who will become infected throughout the world in the 1990s, that is, by the end of the century. Estimates of the size of the currently HIV-infected population are essential indicators of the pandemic's growth potential. According to Robert T. Earickson (1990), epidemiological and mathematical models of the AIDS pandemic can predict the short-term diffusion of HIV in countries or cities for which there are reliable prevalence data. However, the task of predicting the size of the various epidemics of AIDS throughout the world is fraught with difficulties. Short-term projections are derived from the use of various mathematical modeling techniques. But as Chin underscores, there is "great uncertainty" in making such projections because of gaps in our knowledge of the spectrum of behaviors that influence the spread of HIV around the world (quoted in *New York Times*, June 18, 1991:C3).

The biostatistician Victor de Gruttola and the physician William Bennett (1989) have pointed out the problems involved in predicting the shape of the epidemic during the next fifteen years. Missing is information about the natural history of the disease and the degree of infectiousness of HIV; we also have only sketchy knowledge of the sexual and other behavior of those who are most vulnerable to the disease[5] Gruttola and Bennett point out that projections of the future course of the epidemic require a construct or model based on this knowledge. Current models are only approximations of reality and have been "overinterpreted." Furthermore, they claim that public health authorities in the United States have not made basic information available to both statisticians and mathematical modelers. As a result of this lack of information, the development and use of sophisticated methods required to assess

---

[5] Estimates of the time involved in the development from HIV infection to full-blown AIDS have changed many times. First estimates were that the incubation period was two years. Then it became four to five years, then seven. The U.S. Public Health Service characterizes the time as both long and variable. The median incubation period from HIV infection to the development of AIDS is currently thought to be about ten years.

the AIDS epidemic has been slowed (Gruttola & Bennett 1988:57).

The U.S. Public Health Service readily acknowledges the methodological problems associated with making projections of AIDS cases. A report on one of its conferences states that

> A number of caveats need to be considered in making projections of AIDS cases. A degree of uncertainty is always associated with statistical data and so health policies are often necessarily formulated with less than perfect data and with data that are stated with confidence limits. Data users need to be aware of these uncertainties. In addition, different levels of data precision are needed for different uses of the data (Second Public Health Service 1988:16).

The report goes on to say that projections of AIDS cases in the United States two to three years in the future are expected to be reasonably accurate, but that long-term forecasts of the incidence of AIDS approaching five years and beyond are less so. This is because long-term forecasts depend on many unknown factors, while shorter-term projections rely primarily on the progression to disease among those already infected. One crucial element necessary for predicting the future is the rate of infection, rather than the actual number of cases, and this is far more difficult to predict.

A report of the U.S Department of State (1992:v) predicts that during the remainder of the 1990s, an additional 36 million people will become infected, bringing the cumulative worldwide total in the year 2000 to 48 million. About 85 percent of these new infections will be in the developing countries, primarily in Africa. The report predicts that the epidemic will spread fastest in Asia and South America, setting the stage for a large increase in AIDS cases after the year 2000.

Other forecasts are quite similar. Michael Merson, in a December 1991 MacNeil/Lehrer Newshour interview, predicted 40 million HIV infections throughout the world by the year 2000. And Jonathan Mann and his associates (1992:10) at the Harvard AIDS Institute predict that, by the end of the century, there will be a minimum of 38 million and a maximum of 109 million adults who are HIV-infected. The upper limit means that more than six times as many adults would become infected during the last five years of this century than were infected from the beginning of the pandemic in 1981 through 1995. No doubt, as we get even closer to the next century, millenarian concerns will heighten interest in projections beyond the year 2000.

The geographical spread of AIDS

During the 1980s, the pandemic was concentrated in sub-Saharan Africa, which by 1992 had about two-thirds of all HIV infections in the world—some 6 million. WHO estimates that 970,000 individuals in Africa had developed AIDS by January 1, 1992 (Mann et al. 1992:Appendix 2.3). A total of some 10 million cases of HIV infection is predicted by 1994 and epidemiologists at the Center for International Research of the U.S. Bureau of the Census predict that by the year 2015 there will be over 70 million sub-Saharan Africans infected with HIV (Way & Stanecki 1991:1).

In the United States, the other epicenter of the pandemic, there were 310,680 cases of AIDS by the end of June 1993 (*HIV/AIDS Surveillance*, July 1993:14). Experts at the Centers for Disease Control calculate that the annual death toll (45,000 in 1992) will rise gradually and then level off at approximately 50,000 a year. Nevertheless, in the next three or four years, as many Americans are expected to die of AIDS as in the preceding eleven years of the epidemic. One million Americans are estimated to be infected with HIV and between 40,000 and 80,000 are newly infected each year (*New York Times*, June 28, 1992:IV5).[6]

Latin American rates are rising in the second decade of AIDS. By 1994, according to some estimates, there will be some 2 million HIV positive individuals in the region. Brazil is said to have between 500,000 and 1.5 million HIV-infected people, according to the U.S. Department of State report (1992:6). In the major city of São Paolo, HIV infection increased sixfold in the years 1987–1990 (Mann et al. 1992). Mexico, second to Brazil in Latin America in number of HIV-infected people, has a still-growing rate of infection. The Caribbean epidemic is expected to proceed on a scale similar to that of sub-Saharan Africa (U.S. Department of State 1992:8, 9).

In Europe, every country has reported some cases of AIDS—with the exception of Albania. (Countries with largely Moslem populations, such as Egypt, have thus far had relatively few cases.) Most European cases, of course, are in the major countries: France, Germany, Italy, the Netherlands, Spain, Switzerland, and the United Kingdom. In 1993, concern developed about the spread of AIDS to Central and Eastern Europe, a region that encompasses twenty-six countries. Michael Merson asserted that, while the number of cases is small thus far, the risk factors are present "in a big way" (*New York Times*, April 8, 1993:A2).

---

6 Chapter 3 discusses the nature and impact of the U.S. epidemic.

More alarming than the accelerating increases in the number of HIV-infected and the number of AIDS cases in any one country is the rapidity with which the virus is spreading geographically. The second decade of the pandemic has brought unanticipated and disquieting changes in the distribution of the infection. HIV/AIDS is now being reported in areas that have hitherto been untouched: Greenland, Paraguay, and the Pacific islands of Fiji, Samoa, and Papua and New Guinea.

The Republic of South Africa has moved from a pre-epidemic to an epidemic phase, according to Malcolm Steinberg, director of the AIDS program of the South Africa Medical Research Council (*New York Times,* March 16, 1993:A1). If prevention programs are ineffective, public health experts calculate that up to 20 percent of the population may be infected by the year 2005 (Ijsselmuiden et al. 1993:1, 10–11).

Given the realities of the roles of international air travel in spreading HIV and of population density in creating a receptive environment for it, epidemiologists and other observers have viewed the teeming population of the Asian continent as a potential reservoir of cases. Indeed, new reports from Asia have sounded an alarm concerning the future. By the year 2000, according to a prediction of the Harvard group, the largest number of AIDS cases and HIV infection will be in Asia. This also reflects the judgment of Jim McDermott, a U.S. congressman and physician who directed the Congressional Task Force to the region. He believes that by the end of the 1990s, Asia will become the epicenter of the pandemic, replacing Africa, and thus will be "host to the fastest- growing AIDS population in the world" (McDermott 1991:1). Two years later, Michael Merson, writing in the journal *Science,* stated that given Asia's population its epidemic "may ultimately dwarf all others in scope and impact" (Merson 1993:1266).

In Thailand, infection rates have been soaring. In 1991, the Thai government and the WHO estimated that 300,000 Thais were infected and that by 1997 between 125,000 and 150,000 Thais will have died of AIDS ("Focus: Thailand" 1991). By the year 2000, from 3 to 6 million Thais—five to 10 percent of the population—may become infected (McDermott 1991:1).

WHO estimates that there are 250,000 HIV-infected people in India, although some reports suggest a much larger figure, perhaps 1 million (U.S. Department of State 1992:8). McDermott refers to India as a "silent volcano" for AIDS; some 5 million people are expected to become infected in the next few years. By the year 2000, in McDermott's judgment, there will be more infected people in India than there are now in the entire world.

Elsewhere on the Asian continent, Myanmar (formerly Burma) is considered a potential locus of infection since it shares borders with both India and Thailand, both of which have flourishing drug trades (Mirante 1992).

In discussing the geographic spread of the pandemic, the Harvard study notes that fifty-seven countries have so far escaped the brunt of the attack, the largest of which are Bangladesh, China, Egypt, Indonesia, Nigeria, and Pakistan. But the editors warn that the global lesson of the pandemic is that HIV will reach most, if not all human communities. They believe that geography may delay the epidemic, but it will not protect against its certain introduction and spread.

Shifting patterns of transmission

The AIDS virus—which seems to have originated in Africa— is now found in all the major cities of the world and in many rural areas as well. Thus far, however, AIDS is predominantly an urban disease in both the developing and the developed world. Although it is found worldwide, it is distinguished by sharp geographical, ethnic, and gender variations. An editorial in the *Journal of the American Medical Association* (Allen & Setlow 1991) underscores that the broad brush strokes with which the pandemic is described tend to obscure the subtle complexities of the HIV transmission that occurs in different geographical areas and population groups.

In brief, the patterns of transmission of the AIDS pathogen vary throughout the world and are continually in flux. The modes of transmission, however, are everywhere the same: (1) sexual relations with infected partners, (2) injections with needles contaminated with HIV-infected blood (primarily through needle sharing by drug addicts), (3) contaminated blood transfusions, or (4) perinatal infection occurring when infected mothers pass on the virus during or shortly after the birth of an infant.

While he was at the World Health Organization, Jonathan Mann categorized the countries where AIDS took hold and spread during the first decade of the pandemic as falling into one of three dominant patterns of transmission. These patterns that have been widely cited in the literature on the pandemic (e.g., Osborn 1990: 404-405):

> *Pattern I countries*, in which the transmission has oc-
> curred primarily among homosexual or bisexual males

and among intravenous drug users.

Pattern II countries, in which the predominant mode has been unprotected heterosexual relations.

Pattern III countries, in which there have been few cases of AIDS or even of HIV.

In the first decade of AIDS, Pattern I characterized the countries of North and South America, Western Europe, Australia, and New Zealand. Pattern II prevailed in sub-Saharan Africa and the Caribbean; and Pattern III in Eastern Europe, North Africa, the Middle East, and parts of Asia.

But the pandemic has been kaleidoscopic, so that the behavior described by the classification has shifted during the second decade. As the pandemic has continued to spread and as new data have become available, it is increasingly evident that countries categorized as falling into one of the major patterns are in the process of transformation. Thus, in the United States, where homosexual–bisexual relations and intravenous drug use have predominated as modes of transmission, the proportions of these modes are shifting, with an increase in both drug use transmission and heterosexual AIDS. In Brazil, the proportion of cases linked to intravenous drug use has been increasing twofold recently, although homosexual–bisexual AIDS is also widespread. In Europe, where early in the epidemic in 1985 homosexual transmission predominated, there has been a dramatic shift. By 1990, half of all new cases in the major Western European countries—and particularly in Italy, Spain, and Switzerland—were attributed to injection drug use. But in Czechoslovakia and Hungary, homosexual and bisexual transmission predominate. Poland and Yugoslavia combine intravenous drug use transmission with homosexual and bisexual transmission. In Poland, according to the Harvard study, the first HIV-infected drug user was detected in 1988, but by 1991, 70 percent of HIV-infected people were drug users (Mann et al. 1992:2).

Although it was useful in the first decade, the WHO classification scheme has become outdated. Stressing the provisional nature of any classification scheme, Jonathan Mann and his colleagues at Harvard devised a different classification scheme for tracking the pandemic, one based primarily on geographical location and thus entitled Geographic Areas of Affinity (GAA).

The new classification is intended to provide "a composite picture" of the pandemic, created by "superimposed images, each of which continues to evolve" (Mann et al. 1992:23). This new geography of AIDS divides the world into ten GAAs.[7] The new classification scheme uses fourteen social indicators in creating the GAA zones. These include (1) epidemiological factors, for example, major modes of HIV transmission, (2) operational–programmatic factors, for example, percentage of GNP spent on health services, and (3) societal factors, such as the annual growth rate of the urban population. The editors warn that even this classificatory system is based on generalizations and assumptions and must be interpreted as an interim classification. The goal is to create a model flexible enough to illustrate changing national, regional, and local conditions while presenting a coherent worldwide view of the pandemic and the response to it" (Mann et al. 1992:22).

The predominant mode of HIV transmission worldwide has been sexual intercourse: some 70 percent of all new cases are from heterosexual intercourse and 15 percent from homosexual (Mann et al. 1992:33). Responding to this worldwide expansion of AIDS, June E. Osborn (1990:404), dean of the School of Public Health at the University of Michigan and chair of the U.S. National Commission on AIDS, asserted that "the virus of AIDS is so widespread that it is unlikely ever to be eradicated, and as time passes the fact that it can be transmitted by sexual intercourse of most sorts is likely to broaden its distribution." The consequence is that the apparent variation in types of epidemic pattern may well be short-lived. "The disease is now everywhere," Michael Merson said in an interview. "We want to get home the point that the AIDS epidemic is becoming heterosexual everywhere" (*New York Times*, July 21, 1992:C3).

The changing sex ratio

Perhaps the most profound shift in the characteristics of the pandemic as it enters its second decade is the sex composition of HIV infection and AIDS cases. As a consequence of the worldwide shift to predominantly heterosexual transmission, women throughout the world are becoming infected with the virus as often as men. Merson, speaking at the July 1992 International Conference on AIDS in Amsterdam, reported that since the beginning of the year, one half of the newly-infected adults had been women. "By the year 2000," he predicted, "most new infections will be in women" (*New York Times*, July 21, 1992:C3).

---

[7] The areas are (1) North America, (2) Western Europe, (3) Oceania, (4) Latin America, (5) Sub-Saharan Africa, (6) the Caribbean, (7) Eastern Europe, (8) South East Mediterranean, (9) Northeast Asia, and (10) Southeast Asia (Mann et al. 1992:869).

A 1992 report of the United Nations Development Programme (UNDP) highlights the seriousness of AIDS among women, particularly in the developing world. The report points out that:

- Women are increasingly becoming HIV-infected.
- In most of the developing world, there are as many infected women as there are infected men.
- Women are becoming infected at a significantly younger age than are men—in fact, some five to ten years younger than men.
- Proportionately more girls and young women in their teens and early twenties are becoming infected.

No certain explanation of these trends is available, but the report gives the plausible reason that women become infected more easily than men—most certainly when they are either young or after menopause. It is believed that women may have a biological, immunological, and/or virological susceptibility to HIV which changes with age.

The UNDP report not only presents data on HIV infection: it also sounds an "urgent alarm." The loss to the world of many of its women would be a societal tragedy. In emotional and analytical language rarely found in a UN report, it makes a strong case for the centrality of women in social life:

Women bring to daily life different qualities from men. Women tend to be the guardians of compassion rather than ambition, of connectedness rather than control, of healing rather than harming, of closeness rather than conquest, of mercy rather than judgement. They make possible the circle of the dance as an alternative to the ladder (UNDP 1992:4).

AIDS as harbinger

In the pandemic's second decade the shape of the future seems clearer than it did as recently as the late 1980s and the appraisals are more realistic. Viewed as a biomedical phenomenon, HIV/AIDS is seen by many scientists as a harbinger of the future, a much-needed object lesson of the inevitability of epidemics and pandemics in the modern world. The Nobel-prize-winning geneticist Joshua Lederberg has warned, as have others, against the false optimism that periodically raises the hope of conquering infectious disease.[8] In 1988, he stated that "we will face similar catastrophes again and will be even more confounded in dealing with them if we do not come to grips with the realities of the place of our species in nature" (quoted in Garrett 1992:826).

In an article in *Science*, Richard M. Krause (1992) calls AIDS the best contemporary example of human vulnerability to the microbial world. Scientists are genuinely concerned, he reports, that another new microbe or a genetic variation of an old one will "go global" in the same manner as HIV. There have been warnings, he points out, that strange epidemics have been occurring in different parts of the world. Small-scale epidemics caused by bacteria and old and new viruses have been an ever-present reality of the last quarter century. During this period, the United States was startled by outbreaks of legionnaires' disease, toxic shock syndrome, and Lyme disease. Epidemics of viral diseases such as the often fatal Ebola fever in Africa, Asian influenza, and hemorrhagic fever in Central and South America are other examples of the threat of mass infectious disease.

Declining interest in infectious disease was responsible for reduced federal budgets for research in microbiology and virology in the United States in the 1970s. This decline in both interest and funding was slowly reversed in the 1980s as the AIDS epidemic progressed. As Jonathan Mann and his colleagues (1992:227–228) point out, there is "a great global lesson" in the fact that the presence of a new pandemic was not suspected as HIV spread "silently and unnoticed." The lesson is that the modern world is "uniquely favorable to global spread of infectious agents." Whether or not new microbiological threats emerge as isolated ecologies come in contact with the modern world, or whether old organisms mutate or extend their range, the fundamental need will be to detect them as soon as possible. The advent of AIDS has shown "that a seemingly obscure health event in one place can become, within a short time, a health crisis at home" (227).[9] Moreover, as the pandemic continues to grow,

---

[8] In 1969, the end of the successful worldwide campaign to eradicate smallpox inspired U.S. Surgeon General William H. Stewart to tell the Congress that it was time to "close the books on infectious disease" (quoted in Garrett:1922:825).
[9] Richard M. Krause has advanced the theory that the AIDS viruses have been around "for at least a century (and perhaps longer in Central Africa), causing sporadic human infection" (1992:1077).

the emergence of many variants of HIV, which is a mutating organism, can be expected (Moore et al. 1992:275).

The fundamental reason for this global vulnerability is that the modern world offers many new "gateways" for viruses. Stephen Morse (1992), a virologist at the Rockefeller University, ascribes the increase in viruses to the confluence of many factors. Migration, urban concentrations, lapses in public health immunization measures (such as those in urban America that have caused a resurgence of measles)—all have led to an increase in "viral traffic." Morse argues that society shapes the milieu for infectious diseases in a complex, interrelated social context that humans alter but do not fully control. The AIDS epidemic implies that it will be followed by other viral incursions. To combat the epidemics of the future, a "science of traffic patterns" is needed, a science that will be part biology, part social science. It is a field of research that is struggling to emerge. Jonathan Mann underscores this thesis in pointing out that the last quarter century has witnessed such a quantitative increase in the movement of people that the world has become increasingly interdependent. "The new globalism means," he asserts, "that viruses and other pathogens, already known but geographically circumscribed, have an unprecedented potential to spread. HIV has demonstrated how rapidly and thoroughly a pathogenic agent can do so in today's world" (Mann 1991a:126). Addressing the French Academy of Sciences in November 1992, the virologist William A. Haseltine[10] referred to the "ever-expanding population of immune-suppressed people with AIDS [which] serves as a launching pad for new, highly infectious diseases" (Haseltine 1992:IV19).

It is this prospect, then, that mandates a continuing global response to the AIDS crisis by the industrialized world. Self-interest as much as humanitarian impulse is the operative motivation. The AIDS pandemic differs from other large scale disasters that assail the world and call for the commitment of resources on an international scale—ever-present disasters such as famines, droughts, civil wars, and ethnic conflicts. AIDS is a disaster on a different scale and of a different order—it is a common threat with common roots—and a calamity the rich industrial West shares with the poor and developing world. As Haseltine (1992:IV19) warns, "the epidemic makes it clear that we are our brother's keeper."

---

[10] William A. Haseltine is chief of human retrovirology at the Dana–Farber Cancer Institute, Harvard University.

2
AIDS in the Developing World

The Social Context

The countries of the developing world most seriously affected by AIDS thus far are in sub-Saharan Africa. Accordingly, much of the social research on AIDS in the developing world is concerned with Africa, as is much of the research reviewed in this chapter. But many of the behavior patterns described and the conclusions reached apply elsewhere.

AIDS is primarily a sexually transmitted disease, and the escalating epidemics in the developing world are principally the result of sexual encounters with an infected partner. In all countries AIDS is also transmitted by the use of contaminated needles in intravenous drug injections, by blood transfusions of infected blood, and perinatally from infected mothers to their unborn children. But sexual transmission is everywhere the predominant mode, and, internationally, heterosexual transmission accounts for some 70 percent of all new AIDS cases (Mann et al. 1992:33).

In the regions of Asia, Latin America, and sub-Saharan Africa, one of three different modes of sexual transmission of the AIDS virus predominates—although all modes occur with some frequency in all three regions. In Asia, prostitution plays the key role; in Latin America, homosexual and bisexual behavior; and in Africa, heterosexual transmission.

Asia: The role of prostitution

One major form of sexual practice is clearly a reflection of both economic pressures and cultural norms: prostitution. (In the AIDS literature, prostitutes are increasingly referred to as "sex workers.") Sex for cash is a conduit for the transmission of AIDS throughout the world. It is important in sub-Saharan Africa and in a growing number of Asian countries, and it is widely reported to be a key element in the emerging epidemics in Thailand and India.

Two dominant patterns of prostitution facilitate the spread of HIV in parts of the developing world: entrenched, indigenous commercial prostitution and the modern phenomenon of sex tourism—international charter flights with sexual gratification as the principal motivation. Edward S. Herold and Carla van Kerwijk (1992) describe the global tourism network that links the sending regions (Canada, Europe, Japan, and the United States) to such popular destinations as Brazil, the Dominican Republic, Kenya, the Philippines, and Thailand.

The Thai economy in particular has depended heavily on tourism in the past decade, and Thailand has one of the most open and thriving sex industries in the world.[1] HIV infection seems to have been first introduced into Thailand by homosexuals returning home from the West and by foreign tourists and intravenous drug users seeking cheap and available sex and drugs. From 1987 to 1989, the epidemic is reported to have exploded among intravenous drug users, who then spread HIV to sidewalk and other prostitutes. Since most Thai prostitutes are said to be either heterosexual or bisexual, their activities provide a route of entry into the broader heterosexual population.

Currently, the principal mechanism of HIV transmission in Thailand is heterosexual sex with prostitutes. Although prostitution is illegal, it is widely practiced throughout the country.[2] This situation has been graphically described by the journalist Steven Erlanger in an interpretation of the role that indigenous prostitution plays in Thai society:

> Thousands of brothels, massage parlors, bathhouses, bars, clubs, teahouses, coffee shops and even barber-

---

[1]   Revenue from tourism represents 4 to 5 percent of the Thai GNP. The government has launched large-scale programs to counter the threat of HIV infection, sponsoring educational programs and undertaking systematic surveys. But debate rages about what to do about the sex tourism industry, a major source of foreign exchange (U.S. Department of State 1992:4).

[2]   Thai government officials estimate that there are 800,000 prostitutes in Thailand; most are between the ages of 12 and 16. From 20 to 30 percent are infected with HIV; in the north, more than 40 percent are infected (McDermott 1991:1).

shops serve as fronts for the selling of sex. Some of these establishments are for tourists . . . and some foreigners still arrive on packaged sex tours, especially from Germany and Japan. But Thailand's epidemic is now a Thai–Thai affair (Erlanger 1991:49).

The epidemic rages, Erlanger says, in cheap brothels in Bangkok and other major cities, as well as throughout the country-side, where 80 percent of Thailand's 56 million people live. Patron-izing brothels is an integral aspect of Thai male behavior. Every day at least 400,000 men visit prostitutes and brothels where HIV infection is prevalent. This behavior does not seem to be class-linked: 75 percent of all Thai men have visited prostitutes, and the clientele comes from all walks of life. It is ingrained in university life. Thai universities, for example, have a tradition in which upperclass-men introduce lowerclassmen to brothels and pay for the visit as well.

Erlanger quotes Werasit Sittitrai, director of the Institute of Population Studies at the prestigious Chulalongkorn University, on the fundamental cultural value governing male attitudes toward sex: "This is a very permissive culture where *sanuk*, or fun is a prime virtue. Thai men think it is their right to have cheap sex" (26). Some of the houses of prostitution that pander to this conception are big businesses that ship women all over the country.

Young women who are prostitutes give a range of reasons for their occupational choice. One principal motivation is economic: subsistence, or the need to cope with a financial emergency or to help family members. But poverty, Erlanger notes, is not the primary cause of such large-scale prostitution. Quoting a Thai government official, he writes that poverty is an accelerator rather than a cause and that the primary cause is the value system of the people. Examples cited are the attractions of city life, the desire to return home from a stay in the city a little higher on the economic ladder, the wish to finance the education of a brother or sister, and a sense of obligation that results from the Thai practice of inculcating in children the sense that they should somehow pay for being born.

In Myanmar (formerly Burma), with a population of 42 million, there is large-scale trafficking in women, girls, and boys for sexual purposes. With the collusion of corrupt police and military officials, young people are brought to Thai border towns like Chiang Mai and are sold into prostitution. Edith T. Mirante (1992), who is the director of an information agency that distributes material on human rights issues and the author of the book *Burmese Looking*

Glass, reports that some Burmese girls who were found to be infected with HIV were executed. While in Thailand, they are "imprisoned in dark, rabbit-warren like brothel rooms, speaking no Thai, the prostitutes from Burma have little chance of escape" (6). They are in demand because they are seen as being "AIDS free." Myanmar has become a bridge of infection, linking the AIDS epidemics in India and Thailand.

Fear of AIDS has become an additional stimulus to the practice of child prostitution. At a 1993 UNESCO conference in Brussels on the sex trade and human rights, physicians, police officials, and social workers reported that children and adolescents are increasingly in demand as prostitutes because they are considered likely to be free of AIDS. Delegates described the physical trauma inflicted on children in houses of prostitution in Colombia, the Philippines, Thailand, and Vietnam, where sex industries market the sexual services of children of both sexes. Duong Quyah Hoa, a physician who is director of a pediatric hospital in Ho Chi Minh City in Vietnam, stated that because customers fear AIDS, there is a high price for virginity and procurers "are going after children 10 or 11 or 12 years old (*New York Times*, April 9, 1993:A3).

In India, a much poorer country than Thailand, the HIV epidemic proliferates in the brothels of Bombay, Calcutta, and Madras. Infection among Bombay's 100,000 to 150,000 prostitutes increased from 1 percent in 1987 to 30 percent in 1990. The percentage of AIDS cases spread by heterosexual contact is expected to increase from 60 percent in the early 1990s to 80 percent by the end of the century, according to WHO. Although there is a drug problem, adolescents are infected mainly through sexual intercourse. Indian health officials fear that the virus will be transmitted to rural areas by migrant workers, who come from their villages to the cities in search of seasonal work; while living in the city they frequent prostitutes (Khan et al. 1991; McDermott 1991).

In Sri Lanka, prostitution was once considered a socially stigmatizing disease; today it is a "viable source of employment for large numbers of people from many levels of society," according to Joe Weeramunda (1990:5), a sociologist at the University of Colombo. The dramatic increase in prostitution is a direct consequence of the expansion of tourism in the 1960s. Heavy investments in hotels, resorts, and guest houses were made by both government and the private sector. Although tourism has declined in the 1990s, the vacuum has been filled by local demand originating in urban and semi-urban centers.

Latin America: The role of homosexuality and bisexuality

Homosexual relations between men were the major routes of transmission of the HIV virus in the United States and Europe during the 1980s, but there seems to have been relatively little transmission to the heterosexual population. However, epidemiologists searching for possible routes of entry of HIV into heterosexual populations have focused on the link between homosexual and bisexual and—ultimately—heterosexual relations. They have found substantial evidence of this link in Latin America and the Caribbean. For example, scientists at the Caribbean Epidemiology Center in the West Indies observed that in most of the territories in the region, AIDS cases occurred largely among homosexual and bisexual men, but as the epidemic spread, the pattern of transmission became increasingly heterosexual. Bisexual behavior enables the virus to move readily from the homosexual to the heterosexual population. In Haiti, by far the poorest country in the region, an analysis of blood samples revealed that HIV was first introduced into the country by foreign homosexuals. The Haitians who serviced this trade were largely married men or heterosexual males with girl friends who considered themselves to be heterosexual. The infection spread from these bisexuals to their wives or girl friends, fueling what became a full-scale epidemic. In 1993 Haiti had the highest rate of HIV infection in the Caribbean—largely through heterosexual transmission (*New York Times*, January 25, 1993:A6).[3] In the Dominican Republic and the Bahamas, infected prostitutes often spread the disease (U.S. Department of State 1992).

Dennis Altman's (1990) report on AIDS in Southeast Asia provides an added perspective on the role of homosexuality. He rejects the thesis that it exists because of degenerate Western tourists who spurred the development of a sex industry. While Bangkok and Manila are indeed targets for tourists seeking sexual encounters, there is also an indigenous homosexual world throughout the region—in Hong Kong, Malaysia, the Philippines, Taiwan, and Thailand—where there are men whose sense of identity is based on a homosexual life-style. In fact, the beginnings of new gay organizations can be found in several places in East Asia.

---

[3] Nearly 40 percent of all homosexual–bisexual cases of AIDS worldwide have occurred in Latin America, and almost 17 percent of them have occurred in the Caribbean region.

Bisexuality is known to represent a significant pattern in Latin America—either as an aspect of male prostitution associated with tourism or as a byproduct of cultural biases against overt homosexuality. In Brazil in particular, bisexuality is reported to be widespread. Richard G. Parker (1988; 1990; 1991), while a visiting professor at the Institute of Medicine of the State University of Rio de Janeiro and director of the Brazilian Interdisciplinary AIDS Association, conducted extensive studies of the cultural patterns of sexual relations in Brazil. He found that the relatively clear-cut distinctions that differentiate heterosexuality, homosexuality, and bisexuality in much medical and scientific thinking about AIDS are in reality anything but clear in the sexual practices of many Brazilians. "While these notions certainly exist in Brazilian culture," Parker writes, "they are considerably less significant than the distinction between the notions of *actividade* (activity) or *passividade* (passivity) in sexual practices—particularly among males. The 'active' partners in same-sex interactions do not necessarily consider themselves to be either homosexual or bisexual" (1988:170). Homosexual activities occur among married men who consider their roles as husbands and fathers to be primary.[4]

Intertwined with the issue of bisexuality is the Latin American cult of *machismo*, which sanctions extramarital sex for males. The cult of *machismo* also serves to spread AIDS by encouraging bisexual behavior patterns: men who might be openly gay in other societies are in Brazil protected from exposure by the *machismo* cult (Gil 1990).

Poverty in Brazil is a significant cause of HIV transmission. It spawns prostitution, which provides a means of employment for men known as *travestis* (transvestites) or *michês* (hustlers), who service both married and unmarried men.

The role of migrant labor in spreading HIV infection through prostitution finds corroboration in the case of Mexico. Migrant workers cross the U.S. border to work on farms and in factories. Separated from wives and girl friends, they live in camps often visited by drug-using prostitutes. Consequently, they may become infected with AIDS and carry the virus back home. While this source may constitute only a minute contribution to Mexico's 9,000 cases of AIDS, it is a cause for concern. Sociologist Mario Bronfman at the Colegio de México, who is studying the problem, has found that

---

[4] The case of Japan is relevant. In Japan most homosexuality is covert: homosexuals are generally married. The incidence of AIDS in Japan has been low (Mann et al. 1992:97).

migration produces many changes in sexual behavior (*New York Times*, March 8, 1992:L3).

Concern over the potential contribution of migration to the spread of AIDS was voiced in late 1990 by the U.S. Congress in a report on Mexican migrants. Economic pressures that force people to seek work across national borders are at work elsewhere in the Americas as Haitians move to French Guinea and Chilean sex workers migrate into Bolivia (Mazur 1991).

Observers find it difficult to predict what pattern of HIV transmission will predominate in Latin America in the future. In some countries, homosexual transmission is well established; in Argentina, for example, the Health Ministry reports that three-quarters of the AIDS patients in Buenos Aires were infected through gay sex or through contaminated needles during drug injections. In other countries, Brazil for example, the frequency of bisexual behavior among married men is rapidly introducing AIDS to their wives. A 1990 study of 5,000 pregnant women found that 1 percent were HIV-infected (*New York Times*, January 25, 1993:A6).

Sub-Saharan Africa: Heterosexual relations

Sub-Saharan Africa, with only 10 percent of the world's population, accounts for two out of every three HIV infections worldwide among adults, 83 percent of all infections among women, and 93 percent of all infected children (Mann et al. 1992: 89). Heterosexual sex has been and is currently the predominant cause of infection.[5] Another major characteristic of the epidemic is the clustering of infected countries. In Central and East Africa, seroprevalence data show that the AIDS infection has spread rapidly in some countries, while others have been minimally affected. The Ivory Coast, Malawi, Uganda, Zaire, and Zambia have been the most hard-hit.

Sexual relationships in the countries of sub-Saharan Africa most affected by AIDS are characterized by high frequency and multiplicity of contacts. On the basis of African data, Quinn and his

---

[5] According to Daniel R. Hrdy, a physician and anthropologist at the University of California, Davis, most Africanists agree that there is no significant amount of homosexuality in sub-Saharan Africa, although there may be pockets of it. As anecdotal evidence, he reports the difficulties in obtaining labor for railroad work in East Africa because Africans are so revolted by the homosexual practices of some Indian laborers that they refuse to work with them (Hrdy 1988).

colleagues (1986) have pinpointed four risk factors associated with sexual behavior that increase the likelihood of AIDS infection among heterosexuals: (1) having many sexual partners, (2) having sex with prostitutes, (3) having sexual relations with an infected person, and (4) being a prostitute.

According to data analyzed by the demographers Bongaarts and Way (1989), the frequency of sexual relations with occasional rather than permanent partners, as well as frequent changes in partners, are important determinants of the size of the epidemic. Demographers have posited another potential determinant of the spread of AIDS: the age gap between spouses. Disparity in age is common throughout sub-Saharan Africa, with husbands generally being much older than their wives. Survey evidence supports the thesis that older men who have been sexually mobile are most likely to transmit infection to their wives. And studies of risk factors among heterosexual couples in Central Africa have revealed that previously divorced women who have had more than one union have an increased risk of AIDS infection.

Another outstanding feature of the African epidemic is the generally 1:1 ratio of infection between men and women. But in certain age categories, women in fact have a higher estimated rate of HIV infection than do men. Furthermore, since as early as 1986 there has been evidence of "bidirectional transmission"—that is, female to male and male to female transmission of the virus, but the latter appears to be more efficient. The higher rate of infection among women leads to an increase in perinatal infections of the newborn and can be expected to lead to an epidemic of pediatric death (Piot et al. 1988b).

One pattern of heterosexual behavior in Africa is what outsiders generally describe as prostitution—sex for pay. The crucial role of commercial sex is repeatedly underscored in the literature on the epidemiology of AIDS in Africa. Surveys of HIV prevalence in twenty-two countries reveal that infection rates among commercial sex workers to range from over 80 percent in Kenya and Rwanda, to over 50 percent in Malawi, to between 30 and 40 percent in such countries as Tanzania and Zaire, to less than 3 percent in Somalia (Mann et al. 1992:54).

A series of investigations by anthropologists, demographers, epidemiologists, and sociologists has shed light on a significant cofactor that seems to predispose some African men to the AIDS infection: the lack of circumcision. An initial study carried out in Nairobi in 1987 by epidemiologists confirmed a link between the lack of circumcision and the incidence of AIDS among men being treated for sexually transmitted diseases. Subsequently, another interdisciplinary team studied the susceptibility of uncircumcised males to HIV infection elsewhere in Africa (Marx 1989). The data from an examination of ethnographic literature by anthropologists Priscilla Reining and Francis Conant relating to circumcision practices among 409 African ethnic groups was correlated with AIDS seroprevalence rates by the demographers Bongaarts and Way. In the capital cities of thirty-seven countries, principally in East and Central Africa, they demonstrated a strong statistical correlation between the lack of male circumcision and susceptibility to AIDS (Bongaarts et al. 1989).

The role of culture

The African epidemic has spawned a growing literature in the social sciences which seeks to explain various aspects of the social context in which it occurs. The fundamental premise of this literature is that an understanding of the cultural dynamics of the sexual behavior that precipitates the spread of AIDS, of the economic conditions that motivate it, or of the sociopolitical events that precipitate it, are essential for developing coherent and effective approaches to stemming the epidemic. Examples of some different analytical perspectives follow.

The Caldwell sexuality thesis. The difficulty of understanding the patterns of HIV diffusion in Africa is highlighted by the contrast between the views of a distinguished Africanist demographer—John C. Caldwell of the Australian National University—and the quite different views of other Africanists. In a review of the literature on African sexual behavior, Caldwell and his colleagues (1989) at the National Centre for Epidemiology and Population Health in Canberra address the problem of the validity of Western interpretations of African sexuality. Their central thesis is that African norms and behavior should not be compared to those of the West. Sub-Saharan African society is an internally consistent society, which they term an "alternative civilization" (212)—meaning an alternative to Western civilization. It is a civilization, they claim, that is very different in its workings, including its sexual patterns, than outsiders prescribing cures or even offering sympathy often realize.

On the issue of the use of the term "promiscuous" to describe African sexual patterns, Caldwell and his colleagues are critical of the ultrasensitivity of a number of anthropologists to its use. However, they admit that this ultrasensitivity is understandable in the context of combating the stigma attached to such concepts. The authors insist that with the advent of AIDS it has become essential to view African sexual patterns in a neutral manner in order to understand sub-Saharan African society and the role that sexual relations play within it. Their review essay argues that "there is a distinct and internally coherent African system embracing sexuality, marriage and much else, and that it is no more right or wrong, progressive or unprogressive than the Western system" (187).

Drawing mainly from recent research in anthropology (ethnographic studies), demography (fertility studies), and social psychology (knowledge, attitudes, and practice of family planning studies), the Caldwell essays examine the distinguishing features of sub-Saharan societies that govern relationships between the sexes. Although the "ethnic map" is not complete, there is evidence of marked similarities among the peoples of East, West, and Southern Africa. The main points of this analysis are as follows:

African social systems, as described in the Caldwell essay, place great emphasis on *ancestry and descent.* The concept of lineage places greater value on intergenerational links than on conjugal ones. Marriage is not seen as the threshold of sexual activities; rather, its importance lies in its role in allying families and clans. The marriage bond is typically weak, and the primary loyalties of spouses are to the lineage rather than to each other. The most important cultural question is not "Are you married?" but "Do you have children?"

Polygyny is still widespread, although there are signs of change in some regions resulting from urbanization. In the African system, the "basic family unit" is composed of a mother and her children.

Chastity and sexual abstinence are not highly valued and there is widespread tolerance of premarital sexual activities.

Fundamental to an understanding of the African viewpoint are the *prevailing attitudes toward sex,* which are rooted in tradition. Sex in sub-Saharan Africa has always been regarded as something that is normal and good for health, and that, if not experienced, might well result in ill health. Moreover, the traditional African viewpoint, views sex as a worldly activity like work or eating or drinking. Sexual acts can have a transactional value; that is, they can legitimately be exchanged for gifts or money. Casual sexual relationships, for example, can provide a source of needed income for school girls to pay school fees and for female employees to pay for job training. This transactional element is also present in married couples. In East Africa, for example, adultery for economic benefit is fairly common, probably because unlike the situation in

West Africa, the women are generally not traders and thus have limited opportunities for earning money.

Transactional sex of this sort, however, is not to be confused with *prostitution.* Because prostitution is targeted as a source of AIDS infection, it is necessary to identify what type of behavior is actually prostitution in the Western sense. Transactional sexual relations of the kind described above are to be distinguished from the commercial sale of sex. A prostitute is a female who sells sex commercially, charging standard rates on the spot on each occasion, dealing for the most part with strangers, and operating from commercial premises or from a brothel that is used primarily for this purpose. This type of behavior characterizes only a small part of sexual relations in Africa, Caldwell et al. report. Demand for prostitution of this type has been created by "migrant laborers, short-term miners, truck drivers, cattle herders, itinerant traders, soldiers, in some locations tourists, and men in urban or mining areas who are unaccompanied by wives" (219–220).

Among the ranks of semiprostitutes are divorced or separated women. On the coast of Kenya, a minority of women opt out of marriage permanently to live independently outside of their home community, accepting lovers who pay for their services in cash. Other separated women who have been divorced by their husbands because of infertility are among their ranks. Fear of infection among the public is reported to be directed primarily toward the commercial prostitutes since they are viewed as indiscriminate in their choice of partners.

Adultery is common throughout Africa. Male extramarital sexual relations are taken for granted and are recognized as an integral part of a husband's rights. Such relations are expected of the normal man. Moreover, the taboo against women engaging in sexual relations for at least a year after giving birth encourages male extramarital relations.

Female adultery is also widespread in most African societies, but it is regarded as being less licit than male adultery. In East Africa, however, adultery by women whose husbands are absent for long periods of time is condoned because such absences would otherwise deprive her of the right to reproduce. Urbanization has brought about changes in the social landscape, among them the legitimization of "girlfriends, mistresses, 'outside wives,' *deuxième bureaux, femmes libres* or champions" (214) who serve as alternatives to wives in polygamous marriages. Although most studies documenting this phenomenon describe this practice as being most common among the educated and more affluent segments of society in the Copper Belt in Zambia, and in Kampala and Dar es Salaam, there is also evidence of its spread among the poor. These unions are almost licit because free marriage achieved by cohabitation is widely recognized through most of Africa. However, these unions are generally of short duration because wives resent them as a drain on their family income.

No picture of African societies is complete without noting the *cultural impact of Christian morality* introduced during colonialism. A study of sexual behavior among adolescents in Dar es Salaam and elsewhere in Tanzania by a team of behavioral scientists found that missionary values have had profound effects on marriage patterns and sexuality. But now even these Western moral values are being eroded by the pace of urbanization. Adolescents from rural areas attending schools in cities often live in crowded rental accommodations without adult supervision and without separation by age and gender—separations that historically formed the context of socialization into sexuality. The result is sexual exploitation of adolescents, especially girls, by "sugar daddies."

In summary, the Caldwell thesis is that in the African system sexual relations are simple and straightforward; they are not fraught with the puritan sense of guilt that is said to burden sexual relations in the West. As Caldwell et al. report, transactions relating to sexual activity have been looked upon in Africa as normal as those relating to work. African societies have characteristics which the modern West, "largely cut off now from its landed roots and either losing its religion or secularizing" (222), has been accentuating. An understanding of these basic values is crucial to the success of educational campaigns to change aspects of behavior that relate to the spread of AIDS.

The Caldwell sexuality thesis provides a context in which to view the reports of other Africanists on the sexual behavior of Africans. The views of a number of anthropologists—Meredeth Turshen (1991a) and Brooke Grundfest Schoepf and her colleagues (1988a; 1988b; 1991), whose articles express both their own views and the views of others—are reported here. They are among several observers of African society who object to viewing Africa through the lens of what they describe as Western cultural assumptions.

Turshen implicitly rejects the Caldwell conclusion that Africa constitutes an "alternative civilization." Rather, she asserts that many of the differences between African and what Caldwell calls Eurasian society are a function of the Eurocentric perspective of most research on Africa; of the use of data often collected many decades ago; of the mostly male, mostly white collectors of the data; and of the unfair comparisons made between African sexual practices and the seldom-realized ideals of the Judeo-Christian tradition.

To the oft-repeated assertion that the African system sanctions a great deal of "promiscuity," Schoepf replies that Africans are not more promiscuous than Westerners. Rather, in Africa "several types of multiple partner relationships are culturally valued in various social milieus" (Schoepf et al. 1991:188). In fact, African societies contain both exclusively monogamous couples and celibate single people.

The Caldwell thesis states that high divorce rates in Africa are a function of weak marriage bonds; Turshen asserts that divorce is keyed to African social and economic conditions and tends to rise in periods of instability. Moreover, she says, divorce rates are no higher in Africa than they are in France, for example.

On prostitution, Turshen points to a European and feminist literature that stresses that the sale of sexual services is likely to be common in societies where marriage is nearly universal, poverty is extensive, living standards are low, educational opportunities are restricted, especially for girls, and couples are frequently separated when men migrate in search of work. In such societies, the line between infidelity and prostitution quickly blurs.

Schoepf and her colleagues also reject the theory of a special African sexuality. On prostitution, they report that many poor women say that now more than ever they need to find "spare tires" (*pneus de rechange*)—men to whom they can offer sexual services when they need ready cash to obtain health care for a sick child or to meet social obligations (1988b:217). Waite (1988) decries the influence of stereotypes of African sexuality based on myths that originated in the missionary era during the colonial period.

Political and economic interpretations of the African epidemic

Africanists Barnett and Blaikie (1992) present case studies in which economic insecurity for women has led to various liaisons with men, creating a focus of infection in Uganda, Buganda, and the Rakai district.[6] In an analysis of the constraints that African states

---

[6] For an African's perspective on African sexual behavior, see Mutambirwo (1992).

face in their attempts to halt the spread of AIDS, Alfred J. Fortin (1990) makes a distinction between the short and the long view of the cause and course of human infections. Although he believes both views are necessary, and he provides examples of both, his major interest is in the long view, specifically in the historical role of Western colonization in Africa.

Fortin states that Western political development "has carved its legacy into the bodies of Africans," and that the health and sickness of Africans "is still mediated . . . by the effects of Western colonization" (222–223). He notes that these effects have taken three historical forms:

- The introduction of new pathogens by Westerners into African populations with little or no immunological experience of their effects.
- The creation of sickness-producing social formations as a product of colonialist development and expropriation of African resources.
- The disruption of the fragile ecological balance among culture, environment, pathogenic organisms, and the human immune system through land use policies and the displacement of indigenous populations.

The Africans' adverse reaction to the African origin theory of AIDS, Fortin maintains, is not so much a substantive rejection as it is "a consequence of the battle between African sensitivities over the historic injuries sustained at the hands of the West, and the continuing self-serving and myopic image that the West has of its own role in the eradication of disease on that continent" (223).

Based on historical data and on social and economic development theory, Charles W. Hunt (1988), a sociologist at the University of Oregon, provides another perspective on the problem of AIDS in Africa. Like Fortin, he advances the theory that the main African social, political, and economic reality is the situation of underdevelopment and the dependency relations of many African nations with respect to the core capitalistic countries. His primary thesis is that this situation of dependency, particularly as it affects health, labor, and agricultural development, has been the principal determinant of disease patterns in Africa. The migrant labor system that has developed because of this dependency has resulted in long family separations that have had serious physical and psychological repercussions. The combination of this pattern of long separation of husbands and wives disrupted conjugal sexual relations and increased both prostitution and venereal disease well before AIDS appeared on the scene. Male migrants were and continue to be exposed to exclusively male environments, and the resultant resort to prostitution has spread AIDS. Sick migrant workers, as well as sick urban slum dwellers, return to their villages carrying disease. According to Hunt, there is little question that AIDS strikes such vulnerable populations. Using various constructs deriving from this theory, Hunt concludes that they explain seropositivity in Burundi, Rwanda, Uganda, Zaire, and Zambia. Data on seropositivity and AIDS testing show that the AIDS epidemic now ravaging Africa occurs most dramatically where there is a concentration of industry and development, as in Uganda, with the resulting migrant labor patterns and attendant prostitution.

Social scientists Norman Miller and Manuel Carballo (1989) provide additional evidence on the role of migration in the spread of AIDS in Africa. Migration is a consequence of unplanned economic development that created new urban environments in the 1960s and 1970s. Migrant laborers, leaving rural areas to seek work in urban areas, often settle in "bachelor towns"—squatter areas or shanty towns on the "septic fringes" of large cities—where, because of loneliness and depression, they may engage in risky sexual behavior. For women, the consequences of the need to migrate to cities in search of work are even more negative. Women traveling to cities generally leave villages where they are well known and have strong family ties; they become faceless job seekers in overcrowded labor markets, seeking positions as waitresses, bar tenders, or casual laborers. Many are forced into jobs as sex workers.[7]

A somewhat different perspective on AIDS in Africa is offered by Randall M. Packard, a medical historian at Tufts University, and Paul Epstein (1992), the medical director of a multidisciplinary AIDS program at the Cambridge [Massachusetts] Hospital Multidisciplinary Program. Their fundamental thesis is that the pattern of multiple sexual relations in Africa is the result of various social, economic, and political pressures and not simply of cultural norms. They see a parallel between efforts to control the spread of HIV in Africa and the limitations on efforts to control population growth. They claim that, under the influence of social scientists, medical researchers have become fixed on sexual mores as prime contributors to the AIDS epidemic, and as a result other, more important factors have

---

[7] For additional insights into the contributing role of migration in the spread of AIDS from urban to rural areas, see Yeager (1988).

been neglected. "Social scientists," Packard and Epstein maintain, "[have] contributed to a narrowing of research and to the development of a medical model centered on the problem of African sexuality. This paradigm has prevented researchers from exploring factors that may be of equal or greater importance" (359). They assert that the sexual behavior model suggests programs in behavioral modification. However, before we spend millions of dollars on this model, they believe, we must have a higher level of certainty about how HIV is actually transmitted. If poverty and unemployment are in fact the root causes, we must in turn address the causes of these conditions. They maintain that background infections and malnutrition are equal or more important co-factors in predisposing Africans to acquiring AIDS.

If background infections do, in fact, facilitate the transmission of AIDS, then the population at risk is not the urban middle class but the more vulnerable urban poor, the authors hold. They point out, moreover, that few studies have attempted to account for the influence of social class on the incidence of AIDS. If, on the other hand, it is found that malnutrition, combined with concurrent diseases that suppress the immune system, are predisposing factors, "then the potential risk group may be very large indeed, and certainly is not limited to prostitutes, truck drivers, and bureaucrats" (Packard & Epstein 1992: 362). The risk group will surely include the rural families from which infected urban workers come and to which they will eventually return.

The role of the military in the AIDS epidemic is stressed by the British geographers M. E. Smallman-Raynor and A. D. Cliff (1991:69–70), who point out that "scant attention has been paid to the historical association between soldier–prostitute contact and the spread of sexually transmitted diseases for the diffusion of HIV in the countries of Central Africa which have recently experienced civil war." Analyzing Ugandan surveillance data, they examine three hypotheses that may explain the spread of AIDS: (1) the "truck town" hypothesis (major roads act as the principal corridors); (2) the migrant labor hypothesis; and (3) the military hypothesis. They conclude that, although the first two hypotheses have gained currency, they do not fully explain the variability, district by district, in AIDS incidence. Although major roads are currently viewed as the principal corridors of disease throughout Africa, they believe that their military hypothesis is confirmed by the highly significant positive correlation between the deployment of the Uganda National Liberation Army in 1979 and the spatial distribution of AIDS cases in Uganda in the mid- to late 1980s.

The military's role in Myanmar in precipitating conditions that are ripe for the spread of the HIV infection is also confirmed by Edith T. Mirante (1992). There the military dictatorship enforced the relocation of ethnic groups. Open warfare and a "scorched earth" campaign in the forests of tribal areas created conditions conducive to the spread of HIV and other infectious diseases.

Barnett and Blaikie (1992) indict both the war of liberation in Uganda that overthrew the dictator Idi Amin in 1979 and the subsequent civil war that brought the government of President Museveni to power for creating conditions ripe for the spread of AIDS. Warfare has always entailed decreased sexual control, they point out, with rape as its extreme expression.

War and its social disruptions can have a strong impact on the epidemic. One attempt, this one to assess the impact of so-called low-intensity warfare in Angola, Mozambique, and Zimbabwe, examined the effect of protracted military conflicts that can be so characterized. These are wars in which open conflict alternates with periods of civil strife, economic sabotage, banditry, and the destruction of such vital components of the infrastructure as health and educational services.

Since the 1970s, low-intensity wars in sub-Saharan Africa have devastated the economies and displaced massive numbers of people. Civilians flee their homes to seek safety near army barracks. At the same time, regular armies and hordes of bandits are on the move. These movements, largely of young men, facilitate the movement of nonprofessional sex workers who function as bridges of infection to the general population through multiple heterosexual encounters, spreading AIDS as well as other sexually transmitted diseases (STDs). These byproducts of low-intensity wars are by no means confined to Africa.

The case of the Republic of South Africa, where the epidemic began only in 1992, provides a social context that combines economic and political root causes. Natalie Stockton, director of the South African government's AIDS program, describes AIDS as a "total paradigm" that includes poverty, violence, and the powerlessness of women (New York Times, March 16, 1993:A1). Unemployment, the disruption of families and communities by apartheid, and the migrant labor system are all contributing factors to the spread of HIV infections. Conflict between the Inkatha Freedom party and the African National Congress is hampering attempts to combat AIDS. Apartheid's legacy of differential access to health care and ideological polarizations among health workers complicate the task of arriving at a national AIDS strategy before a political settlement between the black majority and the white minority is reached (Ijesselmuiden et al. 1993:1, 10–11).

The Health Context

The role of other diseases

The spread of AIDS is facilitated by a number of diseases collectively called "co-factors"; they weaken the immune system and predispose individuals to succumbing to the HIV pathogen.

Particularly in the developing countries, sexually transmitted diseases (STDs) and tuberculosis (TB) aggravate HIV infection and are, in turn, aggravated by HIV infection. A report by Nancy Berezin (1992) in *AIDS in the World* provides a useful overview of the links between HIV and other STDs. The number of new infections of STDs is much larger than the number of new HIV infections, Berezin reports. Each year, more than 250 million new cases of STD infections occur throughout the world. Syphilis, gonorrhea, and the so-called second-generation STDs such as chlamydia, genital herpes, human papillomas, and hepatitis B are both endemic and epidemic throughout the developing world. They are also considered a major factor in the susceptibility of people to acquiring and developing HIV infection.

Numerous studies have linked STDs as biological co-factors with HIV, particularly to those diseases that cause genital ulcers (chancroid, herpes, syphilis). The interaction of these diseases with HIV infection is bidirectional. Their presence fosters HIV infection, and, conversely, when HIV infection has already occurred, it may cause more severe manifestations of the newly introduced STD disease. The presence of conventional STDs is estimated to increase the risk of sexual HIV transmission by as much as ten to one hundred-fold for a single act of intercourse (Merson 1993:1266).

Although STD is the traditional public health term for a sexually transmitted disease or infection, a new nomenclature— sexually transmitted infections (STI)—is being used in order to encompass AIDS. The majority of STIs, such as HIV/AIDS, do not result from contact with partners who are obviously diseased but with those who have barely noticed or subclinical infections.

The social factors that facilitate this interaction in developing countries, Berezin stresses, are related to the rural-to-urban migration of young men between the ages of 20 and 40, who have been uprooted from traditional family settings and have adopted more casual sexual habits in urban settings. Their presence serves as a magnet for commercial sex workers.

Other reports corroborate this analysis. In India, according to a report of the Indian Health Organization (Khan et al. 1991), 90 percent of the prostitutes in Bombay were found to have one STD, 50 percent have two or more, and 70 percent have genital ulcers. Another possible co-factor, according to the Indian Council for Medical Research, is cervical cancer. Indian women are very vulnerable to this disease, with 90,000 new cases reported annually.

In another report in *AIDS in the World,* Ramnik J. Xavier (1992:148) refers to the relationship of tuberculosis to AIDS as "a dangerous synergy." The dynamics of the pandemic cannot be understood without considering the nature of this interaction. It is synergistic: that is, the combined effect of the two diseases is greater than the total of their separate effects. "HIV multiplies the problems of tuberculosis for individuals and entire communities," writes Xavier, adding that it complicates both the management and course of HIV infection. The linking of these two diseases is having a dramatic impact, particularly in the developing world, where, according to a 1990 WHO estimate, three-quarters of the 1.7 billion people who have TB live. In sub-Saharan Africa, an epidemic of tuberculosis is growing alongside the HIV/AIDS epidemic. Xavier points out that until a few years ago, TB was considered a stable, endemic health problem, but now—in tandem with AIDS—it is rampant. The situation is complicated further by the emergence of more virulent strains of tuberculosis called multidrug-resistant tuberculosis (MDR TB), which poses an alarming new threat to public health programs. Piot et al. (1988a) note that patients with AIDS who contract tuberculosis have a higher rate of infection, reinfection, and reactivation.

The use of contaminated needles

The reuse of needles and syringes is prevalent throughout many areas of the developing world. Pascal James Imperato (1988) calls attention to the fact that in sub-Saharan Africa, the use of improperly sterilized needles and the reuse of syringes, which can contribute to the spread of AIDS, is widespread. Mirante (1992) notes that in Myanmar even trained nurses and doctors use only boiling water to sterilize syringes and drip needles.

Aside from the lack of effective equipment for sterilizing, another factor that can enhance the danger of HIV infection from unsterile needles is culture-driven: widespread popular beliefs in the benefits of injections. In Burma, for example, so-called injection doctors travel from village to village, giving vitamin shots with unsterile syringes (Mirante 1992). In Haiti, *piquristes* (native practitioners) dispense injections and often administer antibiotics (Imperato 1988). In Brazil, according to anthropologist Nancy Flowers (1988), the local pharmacist in rural areas of the northeast and the frontier may be the only person who administers first aid, gives injections, and prescribes drugs. Hrdy (1988), a physician and an anthropologist, also reports the belief of many researchers that "injection doctors" may be responsible for spreading some of the AIDS infection in Africa.

Faith in the universal benefits of injections persists among Hispanic immigrants to the United States. A study of Latinos in San Francisco revealed the popularity of self-administered vitamin injections. Not only do people not realize the danger of HIV infection through the use of unsterile needles: they feel that injecting vitamins will help protect them from acquiring AIDS ("Newsbriefs: United States" 1992).

A study in Kinshasa found that injections are often administered to all infants and children and that mothers consider them to be essential to any cure (cited in Packard & Epstein 1992:363). Injections are often administered in dispensaries by untrained personnel or by traditional healers using previously used needles. Children are also given blood transfusions by injection when they are suffering from malaria-induced anemia. "The view that injections represent the most effective form of therapy," the authors conclude, "is clearly widespread in Africa" (363).

The precise role that drug addiction plays in spreading HIV infection in the developing world has not been documented, but its potential for spreading the virus through the use of shared contaminated needles looms large. In Myanmar, for example, as Mirante reports, there has been a large increase in heroin use, among both laborers and students. (Myanmar is the world's largest producer of opium, from which heroin is abstracted, and heroin can be bought openly.) The frontier areas of Myanmar—with China, India, and Thailand—are becoming "bridges" for HIV infection, spread by both prostitution and heroin trafficking.

The medical use of contaminated blood

The shortage of safe blood supplies for transfusions is a major problem in the developing world. In Brazil, Flowers (1988) reports that 9 percent of the AIDS cases in 1986 and 1987 came from transfusions with infected blood. In Myanmar, little or no screening of blood for transfusions is done even in large city hospitals (Mirante 1992). In the Philippines, 80 percent of the blood supply is not tested at all ("Focus: Philippines" 1991). Throughout the developing world, poverty and the lack of adequate blood-bank systems combine to create hazardous situations. Professional blood donors provide over half of the blood used in Indian hospitals. Not only hospitals but also—until recently—many pharmaceutical companies purchased blood. One study concluded that 80 percent of Bombay's blood sellers are HIV-infected ("Indian Blood Banks" 1991). In Brazil, according to Goldsmith (1988), poverty is so rampant that the selling of blood to unlicensed blood banks for money or for food is common. And in Mexico, where nearly half of all blood used is purchased blood, contaminated transfusions reached such crisis proportions that the government prohibited the buying and selling of blood (Carovano 1987).

The pressing need for, as well as the abuse of, blood transfusions in developing countries is a cause of much worry among epidemiologists. Both Tarantola (1988) and Cordeiro (1988) express concern about the overuse of transfusions in Africa and Latin America because of the high seroprevalence rates among donors.

Fleming (1988) sums up the situation in equatorial Africa as "grim" because of the large number of patients requiring transfusions and the inadequacy of most laboratories that screen for the HIV virus. In describing the magnitude of the worldwide demand for blood, he points out that some 500 million people throughout the developing world are exposed to malaria, another 450 million to hookworm, and about 150,000 infants are born each year with sickle cell disease (120,000 of whom are Africans). Hospitals in Africa make heavy demands for blood in obstetrical cases because of malnutrition, the presence of complicating infections, or the immaturity of the mothers. Moreover, badly maintained roads and heavy traffic in some areas of Africa cause spectacular traffic accidents with multiple victims—further aggravating the demand for blood. As illustration, Fleming notes that well-staffed hospitals in Africa require roughly three times as much blood as comparable hospitals in the United Kingdom.

The Impact of AIDS on Development

A recurrent theme in writings about the AIDS pandemic is that the full measure of its impact transcends the actual number of cases and reveals itself in the nature and severity of a range of long-term social and economic consequences. These consequences are particularly serious for developing countries. Moreover, according to the U.S. Department of State (1992) report on AIDS, the developing countries, lacking the industrializing countries advantages, will be far more vulnerable. The disease will certainly bring about fundamental changes in the social and economic structure of the countries where it is widespread. Moreover, in spite of AIDS-related mortality, the pandemic will not alleviate problems stemming from rapid population growth. Development policies of the last few decades may be undercut or reversed, and donors will feel obliged to reexamine their assistance policies to determine whether to direct their aid to—or away from—AIDS-ridden countries.

Analyzing the pandemic as a development issue, the United Nations Development Program (1991:2) stated that "just as a stone thrown into a pond will create ripples that reach to the farthest edges, . . . so too will the effects of HIV infection be experienced at all social, cultural and economic levels."

Arthur Brown (1988) of the UNDP believes that the poorest countries in the world—that is, those least able to cope with the consequences of AIDS— will be the ones hardest hit by rising death rates in the early 1990s. The economic and social impact will be devastating, he predicted, resulting in declining gross national product rates, the necessity to rethink development priorities, and the deferral or possible elimination of vitally needed development programs.

Looking at the implications of AIDS for the future of the developing countries, Gerald Desmond (1989:5), secretary of the United Nations Standing Committee on AIDS, stated in an interview that "twenty years down the road the epidemic probably will be much more serious—in human terms, in social and economic terms—in the Third World countries than in the industrial world. . . . The disease will have an enormous effect on . . .   attempts to grow economically." The industrialized world, according to Desmond, hasn't realized the full impact of this new dilemma, having been inured to frequent disasters in the developing world, such as famine, drought, and fleeing refugees. But realization may come when the governments of industrialized countries perceive that their efforts to assist developing countries over the past forty years may be seriously undermined by AIDS. Fleming et al. (1988) specify that the pandemic consists of a wide range of social, medical, economic, demographic, and political issues, whose profundity and long term implications call for urgent consideration and action. For Kenneth Prewitt (1988:xi), a political scientist who wrote the foreword to Miller and Rockwell's AIDS in Africa, the impact on development in the affected countries of Africa is "a triple disaster. There is the tragedy of the disease itself, the human suffering, and death. There are the multiple ways in which AIDS complicates the already daunting development problems facing the continent and threatens to reverse hard-won advances." Finally, Prewitt states, "the special characteristics of AIDS—its mysterious origins, its resistance to biomedical treatment, its association with social deviance and its hint of exotic behavior—provide a ready justification for those who would just as soon not be bothered by Africa, its need for international aid, and its developmental difficulties."

The 1992 report of the U.S. Department of State notes that it is hard to conceive of a developing country with both a serious AIDS problem and a thriving economy. Economic assistance will become less effective; generating private enterprise activity and foreign investment will be more difficult; and a growing proportion of economic assistance funds will be channeled to the pandemic.

At present, most countries in East and Central Africa have exhausted their commercial credit facilities. The region is greatly dependent on foreign aid and on international lending agencies. AIDS will act to discourage private investors and there is some evidence that it may already be frightening off foreign businessmen who want to avoid the high medical costs associated with the disease. (Businesses in Africa traditionally assume the costs of medical care for their employees.) Some African economies will undoubtedly be stunted by AIDS; foreign investment in Africa may dry up almost entirely; and foreign companies may reduce their operations substantially out of fear for the health of their personnel and in recognition of the worsening performance of African economies.

A similar future may be in store for Thailand. McDermott (1991:4) points out that the Thai economy flourished during the last few years of the 1980s and the beginning of the 1990s, becoming a model for other developing country economies. Yet this model economy may soon be devastated by AIDS during the next decade. "AIDS may cost Thailand $10 billion in lost labor productivity," he concludes.

Impact on development plans

According to the UNDP, the HIV pandemic will force a fundamental rethinking of development priorities in developing countries. The modalities currently used include various kinds of social investments, such as public lending for low cost housing, the creation of new employment opportunities, and investments in education. The viability of these objectives will be questioned as illness and death take their toll, affecting the ability of people to repay and depleting the tax base of these precarious economies. The necessity of spending on a national level to cope with the rising toll of epidemics and the expansion of AIDS prevention campaigns may result in the withdrawal and reallocation of investments in the productive sectors of the economy.

Human development, the UNDP stresses, is a vital aspect of national development. Education and training play a crucial role throughout the spectrum of social, technical, and economic planning. The AIDS pandemic will further erode the capacity of developing countries to plan, manage, and implement development programs essential in achieving a modicum of independence and decent living standards. Jill Armstrong (1991), an economist at the World Bank, notes that the countries of sub-Saharan Africa—among the poorest in the world—have discovered that AIDS is not solely a health issue. It has threatened the economic and social fabric of their societies and has raised serious questions about the development process itself.

The U.S. Department of State report (1992:4) speculates that AIDS could ruin a nation's strategy of higher education. Policymakers will face the grim question of why governments should spend money on specialized training programs for young people who are likely to die before the investment can be recouped. "This consideration," the report notes, "applies not only to those who are infected, but also to the entire cohort of people *likely* to become so."

Impact on urbanization

Thus far, AIDS in Africa has been primarily an urban disease, although in Tanzania and Uganda some rural communities have been devastated. Although the majority of Africans live in rural areas, there is extensive migration of young adults back and forth between cities and villages. Moreover, some of the urbanized places in Africa are the fastest growing areas in the world.

In a U.S. Bureau of the Census report (Way & Stanecki 1991) projecting the demographic impact of AIDS in sub-Saharan Africa, the authors describe how urbanization has been a dynamic force in developing societies.[8] The migration of young adults from rural areas—those who are more ambitious and better educated than

---

[8] The authors are Peter O. Way, a demographer, chief of the Health Studies Branch of the Center for International Research, U.S. Bureau of the Census, and Karen Stanecki, a statistician with the Census Bureau's International Statistical Program Center.

their contemporaries who remain at home—has been a central factor in the economic growth and vitality of African cities. However, it is these same young adults, without family ties, who are most likely to have multiple sexual partners, and it is this group that was the earliest target of HIV infection. The advent of AIDS may decrease migration as rural populations become increasingly fearful of cities as "AIDS death traps." In urban areas, deaths from AIDS are expected to double the number of total deaths in the next quarter-century.

Impact on the labor force

A key aspect of the AIDS pandemic is the demographic selectivity of the disease. All over the world it strikes at the most economically productive segment of the population: young workers, who represent one of the few economic assets of the developing world. Since the resources of capital (as a substitute for labor) are limited, AIDS has a greater economic impact in the developing than in the developed world. The extent of illness and death from the disease has the potential of depleting critical segments of the labor force in agriculture, industry, transport, and government. Migrant labor—a positive factor in development—has already been diminished. The transport industry, which is essential for knitting markets together, has now become instrumental in spreading the HIV virus. Single males who are truck drivers, sailors, river pilots, and other transport employees have relatively high rates of infection (UNDP 1991; Way & Stanecki 1991).

AIDS is a great threat to the labor force because the years of highest economic activity coincide with the years of highest infection rates. As the U.S. Department of State report (1992) points out, workers begin succumbing to the disease just as they finish their education or apprenticeships.

Key industries in African countries, such as mining in the Copper Belt of Zambia, may be severely crippled by manpower losses. The financial drain of treating affected employees can be disastrous (Heise 1989). Many developing nations have a single major industry: in the countries of Central Africa, copper mining yields 90 percent of export earnings but employs only 6 percent of the labor force. Since over one-third of these workers are in skilled positions such as equipment operation, engineering management, and accounting, the vulnerability of the industry to AIDS is apparent. It takes about ten years to train a mining engineer, and there are few opportunities to obtain replacements from abroad. African countries cannot afford to import or purchase either high-priced sophisticated equipment or skilled expatriates (Desmond 1989).

The loss of workers in animal husbandry, particularly in countries afflicted by drought, increases the risk of food shortages and famines. As more workers are affected, the skills and experience they represent become progressively more difficult to replace. Thus, the indirect economic impact of AIDS in developing countries may well exceed its direct financial costs. In countries where the bulk of agricultural production depends on small plots, shortages of able-bodied adults will diminish production. One social consequence is that child labor may be increased.

Opinions vary on how much AIDS has affected different segments of the population. Studies of Uganda and Zaire have found that businessmen and better educated males are at the greatest risk of infection. Osborn (1990:419) refers to the "disproportionate involvement of young men from the advanced and educated elites, to whom the mantle of leadership was to have been passed." Torrey et al. (1988), referring to the high HIV seroprevalence in urban areas, point out that these are the centers of economic development that have attracted the people who run modern services (although they may not necessarily be the most educated). As an example, they cite the high infection rates among hospital personnel in Kinshasa.

The 1992 U.S. State Department report, noting that elites in Africa have greater access to travel and often have multiple sex partners as well, concludes that their depletion through AIDS will have negative consequences for filling skilled jobs. Furthermore, AIDS can ruin a nation's strategy of higher education. As noted earlier, policymakers will have to explain why money should be spent to train people when the best trained people are likely to die before the cost of their training can be recouped.

The particular vulnerability of the best trained people to AIDS has been termed the "hollowing out" of the elite. The anthropologist Francis Conant (1988:150) has voiced a dissenting opinion, however. He doubts that AIDS has led to a reduction in the ranks of the elite in governmental, professional, and commercial occupations. He believes that fears of this reduction "overlook the robustness of the elite cadres in Africa and the capability of the educational system to provide replacements." Zalduondo et al. (1990:439) note that "despite the attention given cases among highly educated or elite men, it is now clear that people of all economic levels and social classes in high-prevalence African countries are at risk for HIV infection." Indeed, they maintain, "there are reasons to expect that HIV infection, like other debilitating and deadly health threats, will be found disproportionately among the poor. "And the demographer Etienne van de Walle (1990:12) theorizes that the reason AIDS is reputed to be "a disease of the elites" is that "because wealthy men have more extramarital sexual partners and draw more attention than the poor, it has caused great concern among the rich."

Whatever the accuracy of the "hollowing out" theory, as William H. Draper III (1991), administrator of the UNDP, has pointed out, the disease affects adults in their economically and socially active years. The extent of illness and death caused by the epidemic could thus deplete critical sections of the labor force, undermine the public sector's capacity to govern, lead to social and civil unrest, and adversely affect every sector of the economy.

Demographic Impacts

A look into the future demographic impact of AIDS in sub-Saharan Africa is provided by the mathematical projections over the next twenty-five years made by the Center for International Research of the U.S. Bureau of the Census (Way & Stanecki 1991). This scenario is a projection of current trends and assumes that there will be no major medical breakthroughs and no relevant behavioral changes. Here are the highlights of the projection:

An increase in HIV infections. HIV cases will increase seven-fold, and by the year 2015 there will be more than 70 million infected persons.

Population growth. Despite the AIDS epidemic, the population will continue to grow, since there will always be an excess of births over deaths.

Age differences. Infection will be concentrated among young adults, with the HIV infection rate exceeding 30 percent in urban areas.

Life expectancy. By the year 2015, AIDS will have reduced life expectancy at birth for urban dwellers by eighteen years.

Death rates. By the year 2015, death rates will be more than double what they would have been without AIDS. There will be a total of nearly 13.8 million deaths annually, and nearly 4.6 million of these will be AIDS deaths. Infant mortality rates will increase more than 20 percent, and among people in their thirties and forties, death rates will be six to seven times higher than they would have been without AIDS.

Demographers and epidemiologists caution, however, that we do not have enough reliable evidence to calculate the effect of AIDS on death rates. Underreporting of the epidemic has tended to downgrade the seriousness of AIDS in comparison with other diseases. Van de Walle (1990:24), however, acknowledging that other diseases currently contribute more to the overall mortality rates than AIDS does, emphasizes that this "is a new problem which comes in addition to the diseases that already existed, and it has the potential to grow until it occupies first place, and pushes concerns about other diseases in the background."

Impact on families

Social scientists have noted that—aside from labor force losses—the most profound demographic effect of the AIDS pandemic is its impact on families. Disruption of families has already occurred in communities throughout the developing world. Families have been scattered, and villages have been abandoned. As Frankenberg (1988) observes, not only the most productive but also the most procreative segments of the population are at risk in Africa. AIDS thus threatens not only the African family but also the very structure and viability of African societies.

Unlike calamities such as famines and epidemics that affect the young and the very old, the HIV epidemic strikes at the young adults who are both the parents of the young and the mainstays of support for the old (Torrey et al. 1988:45). Referring to the traditional African social structure, Torrey et al. ask: "How will the extended families of Africa and the traditional village societies adjust to the shift in the responsibilities of the young and the old?"[9]

The key aspect of the impact of AIDS on family structure in African societies is the vulnerability of women. It is believed that 3 million women will develop AIDS in the 1990s, 80 percent of whom will be sub-Saharan Africans (Nyonyintono 1992). These women will die earlier than men will, because on the average they will contract HIV at an earlier age. Therefore, since an infected mother may leave a number of surviving children with no one to care for them, the

---

[9] Expert opinions differ as to how AIDS will affect population growth. Mathematical projections made by the Center for International Research of the U.S. Census Bureau—based on epidemiological and demographic data from sub-Saharan Africa—indicate that over the next twenty-five years population growth will continue because of the excess of births over deaths, regardless of deaths from AIDS. On the other hand, estimates by an interdisciplinary team drawn from the Census Bureau, the Los Alamos National Laboratory, and the University of Illinois, conclude that by the year 2015, deaths from AIDS could reduce the population of sub-Saharan Africa by as much as 50 million (*Science*, Research News, April 19, 1991; Way & Stanecki 1991).

integrity of the African family will be threatened, if not destroyed (Way & Stanecki 1991). Inasmuch as women are the mainstay of food production in rural areas, their vulnerability has additional socioeconomic implications (Armstrong 1991).

Traditionally, Africans have relied on the extended family network to care for orphans and the ill. With growing numbers of women becoming ill and dying young, those still unaffected will become, in turn, increasingly the caretakers of the sick. These caring traditions will be strained to the maximum. Beer et al. (1988) have pointed out what these deaths will mean for grandmothers:

> Where both parents and some infants are terminally ill [and] where there are no adequate medical, hospice or counselling facilities, the grandmother will be required over a long terminal period to nurse patients suffering from a disease which is unfamiliar, and whose symptomatology is still unaccounted for, and for which local traditional remedies have no application and no effect. It is a disease for which the grandmother may have no access to advice on treatment or prognosis. She will herself be at risk and perhaps afraid. She will have little or no knowledge of prophylaxis, either for herself or the surviving infants. [She] will have to become the wage earner or food producer (Beer et al. 1988:172).

According to Nyonyintono (1992),[10] little is known about how extended families in Africa function today. This raises the question of whether grandparents and other close relatives can in fact deal with the obligation to raise so many children. The question is: who enforces the norms of obligation?

Barnett and Blaikie (1992) have conducted a number of studies in the Rakai district of Uganda. In Chapter 6 of their book, they present a schematic model based on their research which represents the stages through which a family progresses as it seeks to cope with the loss of family members and their assigned socio-economic roles. Given the centrality of the household in African society, the infectivity of HIV, the possibility that several family members may be afflicted serially, and the fact of incremental deterioration over a period of some five years before death occurs— given all these interactive conditions, the impact of the AIDS

---

[10] Namuli Nyonyintono is an official of World Vision International, a nongovernmental organization in Uganda working on AIDS prevention projects throughout the country.

epidemic is qualitatively different from that of other diseases or catastrophic events.

Impact on children

Deaths among children from AIDS are rapidly negating gains made by child survival programs in recent years. The sheer number of AIDS orphans threatens to overwhelm the family system in some heavily affected regions, particularly when several members of the same family (brothers, sisters, cousins) die in quick succession.[11]

According to estimates of the Global AIDS Programme (*Science*, April 19, 1992), there will be some 10 million orphans in the world in the next decade as a consequence of the pandemic. In Central and East Africa alone, from 6 to 10 percent of all children under age 15 will become orphans because of AIDS. In Uganda, some 115,000 children have already been orphaned by the epidemic (Alden et al. 1991).[12] The children who are not infected will need to be educated and socialized. For those orphans who are themselves infected, the prospects are grim because many relatives will not want to care for them. Assistance programs for orphans in Africa are small-scale and of an emergency nature. In Uganda, some agencies—mostly nongovernmental—provide a system of orphan registration and take care of basic needs. But the problem is a long-term one for which funds are scarce.

Impact on Health Care and Public Health Programs

The most immediately discernible consequences of the AIDS epidemic in the developing world are the burdens it places on health care systems. The nature of the disease is responsible for hospital overcrowding; AIDS-induced infections often require repeated hospitalization.[13] In some African cities, hospitals are overwhelmed by having to provide palliative care for patients who consume scarce material and personnel resources. Heise (1989) reports that some hospitals also have desperate shortages of hospital beds, particularly in Central Africa, Haiti, and Brazil, where a preference is given to patients with curable diseases. A system of triage is already in

---

[11] For a report on patterns of coping with orphans in Buganda, see Chapter 7 of Barnett and Blaikie (1992).
[12] The so-called Alden Report, "Managing Uganda's Orphan Crisis," is a detailed study commissioned by the U.S. Agency for International Development.
[13] Studies in several urban areas in Africa show that a large proportion of all hospital patients are suffering from AIDS (Way & Stanecki 1991).

place.

Stressing that the cost of caring for patients in Africa is compounded by the inadequacies of primary care facilities and the shortage of space in large city hospitals, Griffiths (1988:115) predicted that "it will take some time before it is realized that without large increases in drug and other expenditures, the best policy is probably to allow patients to die as comfortably as possible at home." This pessimistic observation is echoed by Zalduondo et al. (1990), who note that providing palliative care to prolong the life of a person with AIDS may actually prevent saving the life of another with a curable condition. This is a dilemma that raises the questions of where the boundary is between treatment and triage, and how and by whom this should be decided. One result of this state of affairs is that in many high-prevalence areas, where the number of infected individuals overwhelms the capacity of health facilities to provide counseling services, individuals who have been tested and found to be seropositive are not informed of their status. Many inhabitants in rural areas in need of health care have no access to it.

As early as 1986, 35 percent of the internal medicine beds in the major hospital in Kinshasa were occupied by AIDS patients. By 1989, seroprevalence admissions in the major hospital in Abidjan accounted for 43 percent of the total. A similar situation exists throughout sub-Saharan Africa. AIDS strains the ability of even the richest and most organized countries of the world; the developing world, with grossly inadequate funds for public health, faces a disaster of a different order of magnitude. Providing treatment comparable to that given in the United States for just ten AIDS patients, Earickson (1990) points out, would exceed the entire budget of Zaire's largest hospital, where physicians diagnose some 215 new AIDS cases each day. In some high-prevalence cities in Africa, where one out of three adults is infected, up to 80 percent of the hospital beds are occupied by AIDS patients (Merson 1993:1266).

To understand the long-term effect of AIDS in the nonindustrialized world, it is necessary to consider what it portends for the efforts to control its spread—that is, its implications for future public health efforts. As Osborn (1990) observes, the competition between AIDS and other aspects of public health in countries in which AIDS is transmitted primarily by heterosexual relations is particularly cruel. Thailand's Ministry of Public Health estimates that during the next five years 60 percent of its budget will be consumed by AIDS-related expenditures (McDermott 1991).

Quite apart from the problem of coping with the current and future influx of AIDS patients, African countries in particular face the prospect of reduced efforts in the entire field of public health. Because of the strong association between HIV infection and chronic diarrhea, for example, public health efforts in AIDS-affected countries aimed at control of the endemic scourge of diarrhea—which victimizes children in particular—are hampered by the diversion of funds to AIDS. Moreover, the long-term effect of the epidemic may well be that hard-won gains in child health may be reversed as more pregnant women become infected with HIV. Heise (1989) observes that perhaps one-quarter of the pregnant women in some African cities—such as Kinshasa and Kampala—are infected and that up to half the children born will die from AIDS. The continuous hard-won reduction in rates of infant mortality that has been achieved in the last three decades—the so-called "survival revolution"—may very well be brought to a halt.

The full import of the direct costs of dealing with AIDS care and its potential impact on public health efforts emerges in sharp relief when we compare per capita expenditures for health care and disease prevention among developing countries. As Miller and Rockwell (1988b) point out, the per capita expenditure of many African nations for these purposes is less than 15 U.S. dollars.[14] In Rwanda, it is $1.60. In Uganda, with a high incidence of AIDS, the per capita expenditure in 1987 was less than $2.00. In Haiti it is $3.25 and in Mexico $11.00 (Haq 1988; Heise 1989). In fact, as the Panos Dossier (1989) notes, annual per capita health spending in many African countries is less than the cost of a single HIV blood test. Simply to upgrade blood transfusion services to prevent AIDS infection would cost thirty times the annual per capita health budget of Zaire (Earickson 1990).[15] A survey of worldwide expenditures for AIDS for 1990 alone revealed that only 10 to 16 percent of a total of $2.6–3.5 billion was devoted to developing countries, which account for 60 to 70 percent of all cases.

These stark economic realities have sobering implications for both current and future efforts to find cures for AIDS. As the medical

---

[14] Ugandan president Yoweri Museveni pointed out at the 1991 AIDS conference in Florence that most African governments spend less that 1 percent of their gross national product (GNP) on health care, or $3.50 per person per year (*New York Times*, June 18, 1991:C3).
[15] Earickson (1990) notes another economic spinoff associated with increased demands on public health budgets. Foreign exchange credits are lost as Third World governments import items necessary to combat AIDS. Long-term international assistance funds are needed to support both control programs and diagnostic laboratories.

anthropologist Ronald Frankenberg (1988) reports, rich countries—let alone poor countries—can barely cope with the costs of rare drugs that may prevent the development of AIDS in HIV-positive individuals. Thus, Griffiths (1988), of the Health Management Institute in Geneva, questions how many developing countries, which spend as little as one or two dollars per capita or even less on drugs, can afford $12,000 per year for the drug AZT for hundreds of thousands of patients.

Renée Sabatier (1988), director of the AIDS and Development Unit of the Panos Institute,[16] places AIDS in the context of other diseases by noting that some 15 million infants and children die each year of preventable diseases throughout the developing world. Without external financial help, a vigorous response to the AIDS threat would mean that other health priorities would suffer. If deaths from preventable causes so vastly outnumber the toll of AIDS deaths, Sabatier wonders to what extent can policymakers in poorer countries justify the expense of AIDS prevention and control?

The AIDS epidemic in developing countries will force tradeoff decisions. Investing heavily in AIDS control programs may hamper economic development, for every expenditure for AIDS means less money available for national development priorities such as clean water, roads, schools, and other pressing health needs (Rockwell 1989). Moreover, dealing with the AIDS crisis will have a ruinous effect on foreign aid to Third World countries. One study concluded that in five Central African countries, AIDS medical care and screening alone could consume all foreign aid allocations at their current levels (U.S. Department of State 1992:12).

There is a tragic interaction between the social and economic environment and AIDS, which flourishes in conditions of social deprivation and chronic economic shortages. This interaction produces what Becker (1990) calls a "downward spiral." As Merson has noted, the socioeconomic impact of the pandemic will be "immense" (New York Times, June 13, 1990:A8). For Barnett and Blaikie (1992:55-56), whose field is development studies, AIDS in Africa differs in some crucial respects from other disasters: "We distinguish it as a *long wave* disaster because the AIDS pandemic does not take the form of a discrete event . . . It is a disaster that is a long time in the making and in which the major effects have already begun to occur long before the magnitude of the crisis is recognized or any response

---

[16] The Panos Institute is a London-based international information organization that focuses on developing country issues.

is possible." For Draper (1991:1), one way to visualize the totality of the devastating effect of the HIV epidemic is to realize that by the year 2000, apart from the estimated 50 million adults who will by then have become infected, fallen sick, and died, another 150 to 200 million dependents will have become affected—"traumatized by the loss of their parents or children, left destitute, families scattered or children homeless." Thus, the cumulative social, economic, and human costs of AIDS are staggering.

3

AIDS in the United States

The AIDS pandemic has thus far had two epicenters: sub-Saharan Africa and the United States. The sub-Saharan region has borne the brunt of the epidemic affecting the countries of the underdeveloped world, while the United States has had more cases than the rest of the industrialized countries combined. Together, in early 1993 these regions accounted for three-quarters of the world's cases of both HIV infection and AIDS disease.

The fact that a common scourge is affecting these two extremely diverse regions—one the epitome of the economically deprived developing world, the other the archetypical representative of the affluent West—serves as a sobering corrective to a prevailing American ethnocentric perception of AIDS. Partly because of the erratic, piecemeal, and inconsistent nature of data on the African epidemic, Americans initially viewed AIDS largely as an American disease (Altman 1986). Despite the documented spread of AIDS throughout the world, the popular perception that AIDS is largely an American epidemic, particularly a "gay American disease," persists to some extent because the media have failed to convey news of its extent elsewhere, particularly in Africa.

A lack of awareness of the nature of the African epidemic is unfortunate, since comparisons are instructive. For Barbara de Zalduondo et al. (1990:424) at the Harvard School of Public Health, an awareness of the contrasts between the epidemic in Africa and the epidemic in the United States provides a sharper focus on AIDS as a global phenomenon. They argue that the causes and consequences of the epidemic in each region reflect the interaction of the universal (the pathobiology of HIV infection) and the particular (the highly variable health and sociocultural conditions of the populations exposed to the virus) and that these contextual factors are of overriding significance for combating the pandemic. The surprise with which AIDS researchers "discovered" the heterosexual transmission of HIV in Africa in 1986, the authors claim, further illustrates the value of adopting a comparative perspective. Thus, highlighting the key epidemiological differences between AIDS in African countries and AIDS in the United States provides a global perspective on the conditions that permit and constrain responses to the pandemic.[1]

Numbers of cases are misleading and are crude indicators of the nature of the two epidemics if reference is not made to the *incidence* of the disease, that is, "the measure of risk made by dividing the number of cases that occur by the number of people in the population that are at risk" (Goedert 1988:35). Rates of infection alone do not convey the whole story, although as Gerald H. Friedland (1990: 129), a clinician who directs the AIDS Center at Montefiore Hospital in New York reminds us, "the statistics of epidemiology are human beings with the tears removed." What is infinitely more significant than the statistics of epidemiology is the manner in which the two epidemics selectively target different groups in the population and affect the social fabric and the social institutions of these two regions. What is crucial is how AIDS affects the ability of countries to respond to other existing assaults on the health of their people. What is important is where AIDS stands in the priorities of these two regions.

As an editorial in the *Journal of the American Medical Association* (Allen & Setlow 1991:1695-1696) points out, each of the national epidemics throughout the world is composed of multiple subepidemics affecting different social groups, each with its own rates, patterns, and trends. Particularly in the United States, as an editorial in the *American Journal of Public Health* (Hinman 1991:1557) stresses, "the HIV epidemic is not a monolithic event,

---

[1] A similar argument was advanced by anthropologist Francis P. Conant (1988), who examined, on a smaller canvas, some of the social consequences of AIDS in East Africa and the eastern United States in terms of how individuals, couples, households, and both rural and urban ethnic groups are affected by and cope with AIDS. "The premise here," Conant wrote, "is that the experience of AIDS in one region is now (or will be) relevant to the people of another region, even though the two regions may be a world apart." The value of an African–U.S. comparison of heterosexual transmission is also affirmed by Allen and Setlow (1991).

it is a number of epidemics with different modes of transmission and rates of spread in different areas and in different segments of society." It is increasingly clear that, in the second decade of AIDS, each of these subepidemics is contributing to the changing profile of the U.S. epidemic.

As the U.S. epidemic enters its second decade, the magnitude of its impact is becoming clearer as are the details of its causation. The National Commission on AIDS, in its report *America Living with AIDS* (1991c:1), underscored the fact that in less than ten years AIDS had claimed more American lives than the Korean and Vietnam wars combined. By June 1993, the death toll had reached 191,824, according to the data of the Centers for Disease Control (*HIV/AIDS Surveillance*, July:12), and by 1994, the toll will have reached 350,000 (1991c:3). AIDS is already the leading cause of death among young men and women in many parts of the country, the Commission noted. It took eight years for the first milestone of 100,000 cases of AIDS to be reached in August 1989. The next milestone of 200,000 cases was reached in just 26 months, as the CDC reported on January 17, 1992, an event that CDC officials emphasized reflects the rapidly increasing magnitude of the HIV epidemic. In July 1993, the CDC reported that by the end of June there had been 310,680 cases of AIDS in the United States, more than one-third of the world total (*HIV/AIDS Surveillance*, July 1993:14).

As is true of the pandemic as a whole, the reported number of cases of AIDS in the United States is undoubtedly much smaller than the actual number. Furthermore, as the National Commission on AIDS (1991c) warns, the number of reported AIDS cases does not accurately portray the scope of the epidemic, since these represent only 10 to 15 percent of all persons infected with the HIV virus. (There has not been a nationally representative seroprevalence survey in the United States—or elsewhere for that matter. The incidence and prevalence of HIV must accordingly be inferred from small surveys and reported cases of AIDS.) The National Commission cites the CDC estimate that approximately 1 adult male in every 100 is HIV positive and that 1 out of every 600 females is infected. The national total is estimated to be at least one million infected Americans: between 40,000 and 80,000 are newly infected each year (*New York Times*, June 28, 1992:IV5). Some 90,000 Americans are currently living with AIDS (Slutsker et al. 1992:605).

Ascertaining U.S. totals of HIV infections is difficult because the data come from small, cross-sectional surveys that can provide "snapshot" views of the problem but that can only be generalized to a national total by making projections on the basis of assumptions. The problem is exacerbated by a lack of adequate data on the sex habits of heterosexuals in the United States (Catania et al. 1992; NORC 1987, 1992).[2]

Shifting Patterns of Transmission

The U.S. epidemic at the beginning of the second decade illustrates the contention of Mann et al. (1992:18) that neither the geographic area nor the societal boundaries of HIV/AIDS are fixed. In any country, community, or social group, current knowledge of the AIDS epidemic is provisional. Nevertheless, the shifting patterns of HIV transmission in the United States are becoming apparent. Unlike AIDS in Africa, which seems to have cut a wide swath through the sub-Saharan population, AIDS in the United States has thus far been largely a disease of subgroups—as defined by behavioral practices that put them at risk of infection. While heterosexual transmission has been and continues to be the predominant mode in Africa, homosexual transmission and transmission by intravenous drug injections are, in that order, the predominant modes in the United States.

The AIDS epidemic in the United States has moved forward in three waves: first, almost exclusively among male homosexuals; then, increasingly, among intravenous drug users; and later, among the sexual partners of intravenous drug users and bisexual men.

Homosexual transmission

During the first decade of AIDS in the United States, gay and bisexual men bore the brunt of the epidemic. A gradual decline in the proportion of new cases attributed to homosexual and bisexual activity has heralded a change in the profile of the epidemic. By June 1993, only 55 percent of the new cases were so attributed (*HIV/AIDS Surveillance*, July 1993:6). Although the majority of new cases of AIDS still occurs among homosexuals and bisexuals, the reduction has been hailed as a significant accomplishment of the education campaigns organized by gay activist groups focusing on the adoption of safer sex practices. The decline has given rise to some optimism concerning the future of the U.S. epidemic (Ehrhardt 1992).

---

[2] For a discussion of the status of social research on sexual behavior, see Chapter 7.

There are other interpretations of this decline. According to Becker (1990), the transmission of HIV infection was bound to decline as risk groups became saturated with infected individuals. The U.S. Department of State (1992) also reports that epidemics typically reach the point where incidence of the disease levels off at well under 100 percent of the at-risk population because some individuals are naturally immune and others avoid exposure to the disease. However, the point of saturation for HIV varies substantially from subgroup to subgroup, and it cannot be predicted with any level of precision.

Writing in *AIDS in the World*, Slutsker et al. (1992:608) report that the leveling in the annual incidence of HIV infection among homosexuals may result from several factors:

- A decline in previous infections.
- A slowing of the progression of HIV infection through the use of antiretroviral therapy and of prophylaxis against *Pneumocystis carinii* pneumonia, an early symptom of AIDS disease.
- A decline in the number of nonsteady sex partners and a decrease in risky sex practices such as unprotected anal intercourse.

Although encouraging, this leveling off should be viewed with caution, the authors maintain. Incidence may be leveling off among white homosexuals as a group, but there is no sign of a decline among nonwhite gay men. In fact, there is mounting evidence that many minority group members as well as adolescents continue to engage in risky sex practices.

A sobering note concerning the decline of the homosexual epidemic was sounded at the seventh International AIDS conference in San Francisco in 1990. Ron Stall, a behavioral scientist at the University of California, San Francisco, citing a survey of 389 gay men, reported on the return of unprotected anal sex among them (*New York Times*, June 22, 1990: A18). Papers at the eighth AIDS conference in Florence, Italy, a year later reported behavior lapses among gays in both the United States and France (Decosas 1991). There is new concern not only about behavioral lapses but also about a new cohort of younger gay men who may never have practiced safe sex (Ehrhardt 1992).

Stall and his colleagues (1992) analyzed the dangers inherent in the reinitiation of risky sexual behavior among gay men. The danger is not only to themselves, but also to their sexual partners. Two reasons are given. Because of the time lag between HIV infection and the appearance of AIDS symptoms, a gay man who reinitiates risky sex is not so much risking his own health (since he may already be infected) but rather that of his unsuspecting partners. Moreover, because of the high risk and multiple partner environment in which many gay men live, if only a few men give up safe sex, they are greatly increasing the risk of the larger population with whom they have unprotected sexual relations.

Heterosexual transmission

In contrast to homosexual transmission of the AIDS virus, heterosexual transmission has been increasing significantly in the United States. In each year of a recent five-year period, the percentage increase in annual AIDS incidence among heterosexuals has been greater than that of any other exposure category. In fact, diagnosed cases of HIV among heterosexuals increased 41 percent in the period 1989 through 1990 (Slutsker et al. 1992:612).

Available knowledge about the sexual behavior of the heterosexual population of the United States as it relates to AIDS was increased by a 1992 national probability survey of HIV-related risk factors among the general heterosexual population—a study known as the National AIDS Behavioral Surveys. Reported in *Science* by the sociologist Joseph A. Catania and his colleagues (1992), the study involved telephone interviews with 10,630 adults aged 18 to 75. Respondents were asked specifically about their use of condoms in both anal and vaginal intercourse and then were asked other questions designed to ascertain their risk of contracting HIV.

Risk was measured by a battery of questions concerning

- Having multiple sexual partners
- Having sexual relations with a HIV-infected partner or with a partner at risk
- Receiving blood transfusions in the years 1978 to 1985.
- Having hemophilia
- Self-injecting with heroin, speed, cocaine, or steroids in the past five years

On the basis of these indicators, the respondents were assigned to a risk group. Between 15 and 31 percent of heterosexuals nationally and between 20 and 41 percent in cities with a high prevalence of AIDS reported a high risk factor. Condom use, however, was relatively low: only 17 percent of those with multiple sexual partners, 13 percent of those with risky sexual partners, and

11 percent of untested transfusion recipients used condoms all the time. The researchers interpret these and other findings from the survey to mean that current HIV prevention programs have to a very limited extent reached those heterosexuals who have multiple sexual partners but have largely failed to reach other heterosexuals who are at risk of HIV infection.

Transmission through drug use

The complex and dominating problem of drug addiction is a major complicating factor in the dynamic of the U.S. epidemic, as it is throughout the industrial world—but not in Africa. HIV infection among drug users can be traced to their sharing of HIV-contaminated needles during intravenous drug injections. By June 1993, intravenous drug users constituted the second largest group of individuals in the United States afflicted with AIDS, behind homosexuals (*HIV/ AIDS Surveillance*, July 1993:6).

There are between 1.1 and 1.3 million intravenous drug users in the United States, according to reports of the National Institute of Drug Abuse. All are potentially at risk of becoming infected with the HIV virus, as are their sexual partners and their children. New York City alone has approximately 200,000 drug injectors, half of whom are estimated to be HIV positive (National Commission on AIDS 1991c:32). In other large U.S. cities, the U.S. Public Health Service estimates that between 30 and 40 percent of the intravenous drug users between the ages of 15 and 24 are infected with HIV (National Commission on AIDS 1992a:9).

Don C. Des Jarlais,[3] a social psychologist, and Samuel R. Friedman (1989), a sociologist, have pointed out that most risk factor studies show that infection with the AIDS virus from contaminated needles is associated with the frequency with which drugs are injected and the sharing of needles with large numbers of other addicts in so-called shooting galleries. According to Goedert (1988), mortality among drug addicts infected with HIV is nearly 50 percent—five times higher than among drug addicts who are not infected. He also suggests that some deaths attributed to drug overdose may, in fact, be a result of AIDS. It would seem then, that if drug addiction can be considered an illness,[4] as many researchers

---

[3] Des Jalais, a member of the National Commission on AIDS, is director of the Chemical Dependency Institute at Beth Israel Medical Center and a professor of community medicine at Mt. Sinai School of Medicine in New York City.

in the field maintain, it can be viewed as a major co-factor in the spread of AIDS in the United States.

Observers studying AIDS in the United States (and in other industrialized nations) see a tangled skein of interactions involving varieties of promiscuity and drug use. These interactions place certain subgroups of the population at risk and are threading into the main fabric of society.

As a report of the National Research Council—*AIDS: Sexual Behavior and Intravenous Drug Use* (Turner et al. 1989)—underscores, sexual behavior and drug use are often inextricably linked. For example, female partners of drug users may use sex in order to obtain funds for drugs. Unprotected sexual activity, both homosexual and heterosexual, combined with intravenous drug use has raised the total of such AIDS cases to 31 percent of all cases (National Commission on AIDS 1991c). In fact, intravenous drug users represent the largest number of heterosexuals infected with HIV, posing risks to their sexual partners (Craven 1988). If heterosexual transmission of HIV becomes self-sustaining in the United States, intravenous drug use will have been the initial source. Intravenous drug injectors are found in every state. Moreover, they are a mobile population, capable of spreading the HIV infection widely.

The appearance of cocaine on the American drug scene has introduced a new complicating factor. Perhaps as many as 10 million Americans have used cocaine. Moreover, estimates from the National Institute of Drug Abuse, according to Craven, suggest that most cocaine abusers have injected drugs intravenously at least once. The implications of these numbers, he maintains, are "staggering." Norman E. Zinberg (1990:217), a psychiatrist at Harvard Medical School, agrees that this change in style of drug addiction can be expected to aggravate the spread of AIDS. He observes that cocaine use has shifted to a different population: it "has diminished in law firms, financial districts, sports, and the entertainment world," but now "free-basing and the smoking of crack" have spread to the inner cities such as the South Bronx, East Los Angeles, and Roxbury. "Not surprisingly," he adds, "these are the same communities that show the highest and most rapidly rising rates of HIV positive."

In the recent past heroin users have been the main group to test positive, but intravenous cocaine use is increasing rapidly

---

[4] The U.S. Public Health Service defines drug dependence as a chronic medical disorder.

among former users of cocaine in crack form. This group, in contrast to the aging population of heroin addicts, is young and very active sexually, and therefore is more at risk.[5] Finally, Des Jarlais and Friedman (1989) note that several studies of drug addiction behavior show that the injection of cocaine is more closely linked to HIV exposure than is heroin injection. They consider these findings particularly alarming because of the inadequacies of current treatments for cocaine addiction.[6]

The Demographic Profile of AIDS

Geographical distribution

Spread across many countries in sub-Saharan Africa, but concentrated in the so-called AIDS belt, the African epidemic shows enormous geographical variability. In contrast, the U.S. epidemic has thus far been concentrated in and around the large cities. Ernest Drucker (1991:52), a social scientist at the Albert Einstein School of Medicine, has provided some data on the New York metropolitan area. In the south Bronx, with a population of some 500,000, 10 to 20 percent of the population of 25-to 45-year-old men are already infected, and other communities in New York City and northern New Jersey appear to have prevalence rates that approximate those of some areas of East and Central Africa. New York has thus become the epicenter of the U.S. epidemic. Los Angeles and San Francisco, Newark, Philadelphia, Miami, and Atlanta are the other cities with a substantial number of cases.

In the early 1990s, however, new pockets of infection are occurring throughout the country. The epidemic is becoming more and more a generalized American phenomenon and less of a bicoastal phenomenon. The number of cases in municipalities with populations of less than 500,000 has increased significantly, so that by June 1993, 16 percent of all new cases were from these smaller communities (*HIV/AIDS Surveillance*, July 1993:5). Thus,

---

[5] An insight into how crack may contribute to the spread of AIDS was obtained in an ethnographic study of the culture of addicts in New York City. Philippe Bourgois found that inhaling the hot fumes of smokable crack may easily result in cracked lips—which then provide an avenue of entry for the HIV virus during oral sex (*Science*, News and Comment, December 15, 1989).

[6] For additional information about the drug culture in U.S. cities, see Des Jarlais et al. (1992).

all the available evidence shows that—as in sub-Saharan Africa—the swath of the U.S. epidemic is widening.

AIDS and gender

The ratio of men to women with HIV infection, as measured by seroprevalence tests, is dropping rapidly; recently, only three men to every one woman have become infected.

There is no doubt that AIDS is spreading more rapidly among women than it is among men. Cases reported as resulting from heterosexual transmission have been increasing dramatically (National Commission on AIDS 1991c:12). Furthermore, among people exposed to the virus, infection occurs more frequently among women than among men. In many AIDS clinics in New York and San Francisco, 30 to 50 percent of all new patients with HIV are women (*Time*, August 3, 1992:34).[7]

Unlike patterns of HIV transmission in sub-Saharan Africa and elsewhere in the Third World, prostitution in the United States does not play a significant role in the transmission of the infection—although in the early years of the U.S. epidemic it was widely feared that it would. The evidence reported in *AIDS: The Second Decade* (Miller et al. 1990) suggests instead that a prostitute's risk of becoming infected is more closely related to drug use than to multiple contacts with clients. Early in the 1980s, perinatal transmission was the major concern because women between the ages of 20 and 39, who made up the majority of diagnosed cases, were of child-bearing age. By 1990, however, the risk for women of all ages had increased and more and more women, the report notes, are confronting the disease.

Women have become infected primarily through drug use. Although the proportion of women acquiring HIV in this manner has dropped slightly, this decrease has been more than offset by the proportion of women acquiring it through heterosexual intercourse. In fact, AIDS case data show that women are at greater risk than men of acquiring infection through heterosexual contact and that the portion of U.S. AIDS cases attributed to heterosexual contact is growing (Miller et al. 1990:49).

---

[7] That women represent a growing percentage of cases of heterosexual transmission may be explained in part by the fact that transmission is more efficient, biologically speaking, from men to women than from women to men.

Both women and low-income individuals of either sex are more likely than other adults to have sexual partners who are at risk through their sexual behavior. Approximately 71 percent of adults with a "risky" sexual partner reported not using condoms during intercourse. Since it is not women who use condoms, this finding confirms that women are relatively powerless to influence the risk behavior of their partners (Catania et al. 1992).

In New York City, with a plurality of the AIDS cases in the United States, and in the major cities of sub-Saharan Africa and the Americas, AIDS is now the leading cause of death among women 25 to 40 years old (Rogers 1992:522).

Some critics of U.S. epidemiological data on HIV infection claim that women are underrepresented. Because the first cases of AIDS occurred among men, their argument runs, the case definition of the new syndrome was centered on the disease as manifested in men. Gynecological conditions, such as pelvic inflammatory disease (PID), severe yeast infections, and cervical cancer (which is more virulent in immune-suppressed women), were not included in the list of AIDS-related conditions. Another criticism is that similar conditions in men and women have been interpreted differently, diagnosed differently, and treated differently. In the early years of the epidemic, women were explicitly perceived as "vectors of perinatal transmission" or implicitly as "vessels of infection" (National Commission on AIDS 1991c: 28).). Thus, underdiagnosis is a significant bias in epidemiological data on women with AIDS, according to the physicians Kathryn Anastos and Carola Marte (1991).

AIDS and age

Because AIDS is a sexually transmitted disease, most cases—in both sub-Saharan Africa and the United States—are among the most sexually active segment of the population, young adults. This is one reason why AIDS poses such a great threat to societal stability: it is young adults, after all, who raise a nation's children and form the core of its labor force.

In the early years of the U.S. epidemic, when homosexuals were the majority of PWIs (persons with AIDS), 67 percent of the reported cases were among adults in their twenties and thirties, according to CDC reports. In recent years, increasing numbers of infants have acquired the HIV infection perinatally, and older adults (most of whom became infected when they were young) are being reported as having the disease; Riley et al. (1989), in their book *AIDS in an Aging Society*, demonstrate how the aging of the AIDS population will accelerate in the next decade as HIV infections become AIDS and as the population itself ages. But in 1993, in the United States AIDS was primarily a disease of young adults.

AIDS and children

Because women of reproductive age in Africa have a much higher prevalence of HIV infection than do similar women in the United States, the incidence of pediatric AIDS is also higher in Africa. The transmission of HIV from mother to child perinatally also differs markedly between developed and undeveloped countries. In Africa, infected women are twice as likely as women in the United States to transmit the infection to their children. According to the demographer van de Walle (1990), this difference can be attributed to the higher fertility of African mothers, the shorter latency period among small children, and the more frequent use of contaminated blood for transfusions. According to May et al. (1990:69), from 30 to 50 percent of all children worldwide who are born with HIV infection will die of AIDS in their first few years of life.

In the United States, children are now considered to be among the fastest growing group of cases. By June 1993, the number of reported pediatric AIDS cases had increased to 4,710 (*HIV/AIDS Surveillance*, July 1993: 9). Substantial increases in the number of cases of perinatal transmission can be expected in the years ahead (Slutsker et al. 1992:614).

AIDS among adolescents

Through March 1993 there had been only 913 males and 388 females in the 13-19 year old age group diagnosed as having AIDS (*HIV/AIDS Surveillance*, July 1993: 10). However, the threat of HIV infection to this age group is growing. The number of teenagers with AIDS has been almost doubling each year, and over 20 percent of all reported new cases of AIDS are among individuals in their teens and twenties—who were infected for the most part during adolescence (National Commission on AIDS 1992b:15).

The majority of young people in the United States report having begun intercourse—without condoms—as teenagers, and a considerable number report some experience with intravenous drugs. Even more significant, a substantial proportion of cases among adolescent boys and young men is related to homosexual contacts. Thus, the adolescent population contains "pockets" of teenagers whose behavior puts them at risk. Those who are already infected are capable of transmitting the infection to their peers. Others have sexual relations or share drug injection needles with adults, which puts the adolescent population at greater risk.

AIDS among minorities

The major distinguishing characteristic of the AIDS epidemic in the United States has been the selectivity of its victims. Members of minority groups have been disproportionately represented since the beginning, with homosexual blacks and Hispanics among the first cases of AIDS in the United States. For this reason, the National Commission devoted its major 1992 report to AIDS and minorities, calling it *The Challenge of HIV/AIDS in Communities of Color.*

The report focuses on four groups: blacks or African Americans; Asian Americans and Pacific Islanders; American Indians and Native Alaskans; and Hispanics/Latinos. In the U.S. population, the largest group among Hispanics/Latinos are Mexican Americans; the others are Central and South Americans, Puerto Ricans, and Cubans. Unless otherwise indicated, the information about minorities in this chapter has been obtained from this report.

By September 1992, blacks, who represent 12 percent of the U.S. population, accounted for nearly 30 percent of all AIDS cases. Hispanics, who constitute only 9 per cent of the population, accounted for 17 percent of all cases. In 1992, blacks and Hispanics represented just under half the males, more than three-quarters of the females, and almost two-thirds of the children diagnosed with AIDS. And of the 100,777 Americans who died of AIDS from 1981 through 1990, 28 percent were black and 16 percent were Hispanic. The death rate for HIV-related causes among black men has been three times that of white men, and among black women it has been nine times that of white women.

Asian American and Native American rates are relatively low, but because of the relative insularity of these groups, which magnifies the effect of infectious diseases once they have taken hold, the course of their epidemic could come to resemble that of blacks and Hispanics. Although data are sparse, there is every reason to believe that three of these minority communities are disproportionately represented among the HIV-infected as well. One indication is that among applicants for military service and among job corps entrants, rates of infection have been found to be much higher among three groups—blacks, Hispanics, and Native Americans— than among all others.

In the initial stage of the U. S. epidemic, AIDS was perceived as a disease of gay white men. While gays certainly predominated, many of the initial cases were gay members of minorities. In 1990, members of minority groups accounted for 43 percent of all AIDS cases attributed to unprotected homosexual contact (Miller et al. 1990). As a result of this initial misperception, coupled with the effective defensive practices widely adopted and publicized by the white gay community, insufficient attention has been paid to minorities. The incidence of new cases of AIDS among white homosexuals may have leveled off in recent years, but there is no evidence of plateauing among nonwhites (Slutsker et al. 1992:607–608). As Dennis Altman (1992:389) has warned, "the myth that all gay men are rich, white, and define themselves as members of gay communities is one of the more dangerous myths contributing to the growth of the epidemic." Moreover, as David Ostrow (1990), a psychiatrist at the University of Michigan, has observed, a significantly greater proportion of blacks and Hispanics have identified themselves as bisexuals than have whites, a phenomenon that has important implications for the secondary transmission of HIV infection to women. Porter (1989:373–374) refers to the dilemma of bisexuals and homosexuals among minority group members who must conceal their homosexual behavior if they are to remain accepted in their communities. They must, she says, "make a choice between their sexual and cultural identities."

Intravenous drug use has played a significant role in the disproportionate representation of AIDS among blacks and Hispanics. The proportion of AIDS cases among these groups directly attributable to the injection of drugs is four times that of whites—40 percent versus 9 percent. HIV infection rates are also higher among drug users in these two minority groups than among white drug users.

The National Commission's report on minorities emphasizes the special toll the epidemic is taking in the black community:

> If one speaks about woman and AIDS, one is speaking about African American women. If one speaks about children and AIDS, one is speaking about African American children. If one speaks about injection drug users and AIDS, one is speaking about people in the African American community. Similarly, if one speaks about gay men and AIDS, one is speaking about African American men, since roughly half of African American men who are infected are men who have sex with other men (1992b:34).

A major point of the report is that despite this disproportionate infection rate there is no evidence that race is a biological risk factor predisposing blacks to acquire HIV/AIDS. In addition, there is no demonstrated genetic reason for this disparate impact. Therefore, the report concludes, the question of why there is such an imbalance in the response to the virus requires a social explanation.

Minority vulnerability is a function of the social context in which these minorities live. They are plagued by overlapping social problems: low income, poor health, drug addiction, discrimination in employment, crowded housing, and inadequate access to medical services. As a consequence, they are more likely than others not only to become infected, but to suffer serious social consequences. Among these are the following:

- Without access to adequate medical care they depend on overtaxed public clinics. As a result, many are diagnosed as having AIDS only when serious symptoms of opportunistic infections develop, and they are more likely to die sooner from AIDS.
- Because of high AIDS death rates among minorities, thousands of children are being orphaned. A study reported by David Michaels and Carol Levine (1992) estimates that unless the course of the epidemic changes dramatically, it will leave an orphan burden of 82,000 children and teenagers—largely offspring of single black and Hispanic women—by the year 2000. Some 30,000 of them will be in New York City.[8] They warn that unless more attention is given to this vulnerable population, a social catastrophe is unavoidable.
- The lack of primary health care services for many people with HIV disease has forced them to look to clinical trials that test experimental treatments. The strict entry criteria associated with the controlled clinical trials for the experimental testing of AIDS drugs have often excluded women, children, drug

---

[8] Sociologists specializing in the problems of aging draw attention to the added burden faced by those lower income older Americans—black or white—who are forced to become the sole providers of care for their adult offspring afflicted with AIDS or for their orphaned or sick grandchildren (Crystal et al. 1989; McKinlay et al. 1989).

users, people with hemophilia, and prisoners. Communities of color have seen these criteria as discriminatory, since the National Institutes of Health clinical trials group (ACTG) has included significantly lower numbers of minorities with AIDS than their proportion in the HIV-infected population at large would warrant. This is particularly true of blacks. Moreover, despite the high prevalence of the disease among women and the possibility that they may require different therapies, the drug trials have enrolled mostly men (Levine 1990b). As a result of underrepresentation, members of minorities have not had access to the experimental treatments available through the trials.

Tragic as this selective impact of HIV/AIDS on the poor and marginalized segments of American society is, in comparison with the developing world it is as night and day. As Dennis Altman (1993:7) observes, while there are great inequalities in the United States in access to AIDS treatment, in most of the developing world "there are virtually no treatments available to which access can be sought."

Prisoners and the homeless

Two segments of the population, whose numbers are growing, live in conditions ripe for the spread of AIDS: prisoners and the homeless.

In an analysis of the impact of AIDS on prisons, Dubler and Sidel (1991)[9] describe the explosive growth in the number of prisoners resulting in large part from the war on drugs. In 1990, one in every twenty-seven men in the United States was under some form of correctional supervision. One million Americans are in prison, almost half of whom are black (Jonsen & Stryker 1993:16). They live in prison communities that reflect the values and ills of the larger society, in settings that are woefully inadequate to deal with illness in general and with AIDS in particular. Prisons are not designed as

---

[9] Nancy Nevelof Dubler, an attorney, is director of law and ethics in the Department of Epidemiology and Social Medicine, Montefiore Medical Center/Albert Einstein College of Medicine. Victor W. Sidel, a specialist in the study of equitable access to health care, is distinguished university professor of social medicine at the Center.

caring institutions and they are ill equipped to deal with a complex illness such as AIDS: the corrections system is designed to segregate, confine, and punish. Health care personnel are the only independent, autonomous noncorrectional staff members tolerated by prison authorities, but programs for dealing with the disease are generally poor. And with the increase in the incidence of AIDS, the authors realize, prisons will become hospital conduits and nursing homes, or even charnel houses.

The treatment of HIV infections in prison, the authors emphasize, is likely to reveal a profound irony in the system of medical care in America: prisoners are the only group in society with the constitutional right to medical care. Indeed, jails and prisons represent a primary source of health care for those poor and minority Americans who pass through the corrections system each year.

Ernest Drucker has provided a chilling portrait of the future in his description of conditions in the prisons of New York State. Because of increased arrest rates and imprisonment for drug-related crimes, large numbers of convicted felons enter prison each year: between 20 and 25 percent of these new prisoners are infected with HIV. Although they have a constitutional right to medical care, "the prison health services are chronically understaffed and have great difficulty in attracting capable individuals" (1991:61).

In their evaluation of the impact of AIDS on New York's prisons, Jonsen and Stryker (1993:17) note that prison infirmaries are filled with inmates in various stages of HIV/AIDS. In most instances, funds for their care must come from corrections system health budgets that are already "strained beyond the breaking point." (In New York State, two-thirds of the corrections system health budget of about $100 million is earmarked for HIV/AIDS care.) The number of prisoners infected with HIV means that there will be "many more prisoners with AIDS in the future" (195).

The situation in California is not unlike that in New York. Most of that state's HIV-infected inmates are housed in a medical facility in Vacaville. Demonstrations outside the prison and hunger strikes within have led to promises of improved treatment and facilities, but in 1993 Michael Wiseman of the Legal Aid Society, noting that prisons have never provided good medical care, observed that HIV has "turned a lot of them into death camps" (New York Times, January 25, 1993:A12).

The plight of the homeless, an amorphous, shifting, and growing segment of the population, represents what is perhaps the most intractable aspect of AIDS in America. As Arno (1991) stresses, AIDS has struck increasing numbers of intravenous drug users, their sexual partners, and their children. Many of the assumptions regarding patterns of medical care developed initially for gay men have turned out to be totally inappropriate for this marginalized group. The homeless represent different HIV-related characteristics: they are 30 to 40 percent female, they include increasing numbers of adolescents, they seldom have medical insurance, and they lack the most basic requirement for survival—access to stable housing.

The Health Context of AIDS

The role of co-factors

In both Africa and the United States, a host of other diseases—particularly sexually transmitted diseases—provide ground for the spread of AIDS. In the United States, there have been increases in primary and secondary syphilis and in resistant strains of gonorrhea (Slutsker et al. 1992). A study sponsored by the Alan Guttmacher Institute in New York City determined that "more than one in five of all Americans, or 56 million people, are infected with a viral sexually transmitted disease like herpes or hepatitis B" (*New York Times*, April 1, 1993:A1).

For poorly understood reasons, sexually transmitted diseases (STDs) are more prevalent among some minority groups than among whites. STD infection rates in general are extremely high among blacks, who accounted for 78 percent of all reported cases of gonorrhea and 76 percent of all reported cases of primary and secondary syphilis in the United States in 1988 (National Commission on AIDS 1992b:32). Similarly, Hispanics accounted for 12 percent of all reported cases of primary and secondary syphilis (43).

The resurgence of syphilis that has occurred since 1985 among these groups in the inner cities is attributed by Berezin (1992) to the bartering of sex for drugs and to the use of crack/coke. The shifting of governmental resources from syphilis control to AIDS control has aggravated the crisis.

The major problem of rising rates of STDs in the United States is related to society's failure to meet the needs of the urban poor and to control the explosion of crack/coke use. The STD crisis affecting the urban underclass "increasingly resembles that seen in the slums of the least developed countries, where acquired immunodeficiency syndrome . . . has been spreading at epidemic rates among heterosexuals" (Aral & Holmes, quoted in Berezin 1992:179).

Until recently, only in Africa was tuberculosis (TB) an important co-factor in the development of AIDS, but data released in July 1990 by the Centers for Disease Control show an unprecedented increase of tuberculosis in the United States, especially in the inner cities. (Blacks, Hispanics, and Native Americans have historically had higher TB rates than whites. Recently, Asian and Pacific islander immigrants have also had high rates because they come from countries with high rates.)

The same deadly interplay between the old disease of TB and AIDS, the newest scourge, is at work in both regions. Experts in the Division of Tuberculosis Control of the CDC attribute the tuberculosis revival (the disease was until recently not considered to be a major health problem) to the AIDS epidemic.

HIV seropositive individuals with weakened immune systems are much more susceptible to tuberculosis and, once infected, become carriers of the new infection into the general population. TB is much more infectious than AIDS, since it does not require body contact to spread; it is commonly acquired by inhaling droplets from an infected person's respiratory system. The disease is one of the opportunistic infections that are deadly for individuals who are already HIV-infected. According to Anthony S. Fauci, director of the National Institute of Allergy and Infectious Diseases, tuberculosis seems to be the only opportunistic infection that can be spread from people infected with HIV to those who are not (*New York Times*, February 11, 1992:C3). According to the CDC, thirty-one states have reported an increase in the number of TB cases among every racial and ethnic group except non-Hispanic whites and American Indians and Alaskan natives.

Fauci has hypothesized that the spread of new virulent and drug-resistant strains of tuberculosis might become as serious a public health threat as AIDS. The battle against the new strains of tuberculosis—multidrug-resistant tuberculosis (MDR TB)—in shelters for the homeless, in prisons, and in city hospitals has been complicated by the fact that they are difficult to detect in HIV-infected individuals.[10]

Numerous outbreaks of MDR TB have occurred in New York City hospitals, involving large numbers of AIDS patients and infecting not only these patients but many others as well. This serious situation is the result of a confluence of factors:

---

[10] Roughly 25 to 50 percent of all tuberculosis victims in New York City are also infected with HIV (*New York Times*, April 26, 1992:18).

- Large numbers of hospitalized AIDS patients
- Growing numbers of homeless people
- The difficulty of diagnosing TB infection in these groups
- Delayed recognition of the resistance of MDR TB to drugs

Treating MDR TB presents a daunting public health problem since therapy requires at least eighteen months, during which time patients must take at least four different drugs. Some physicians, nurses, and technicians at urban hospitals have been infected, underscoring the need for infection control measures to prevent further spread (*New York Times*, August 1, 1992:1, 9; Slutsker et al. 1992; Xavier 1992).

On January 9, 1993, the New York City Health Department adopted strict regulations permitting the detention of TB patients who fail to complete the full course of proscribed treatment on their own. The move was intended to curb the spread of TB and its drug-resistant strains; curing most strains of TB can take from six months to two years. The new quarantine measures are intended to ensure that patients who have ceased taking prescribed medications after their release from the hospital will continue their medication until they are completely cured. The patients detained in the hospitals will be under guard (*New York Times*, January 10, 1993:1, B3).

The safety of the blood supply

Africa faces a continuing problem in providing transfusions free of HIV infection, coupled with a need for blood products which far exceeds that of the industrial world (Sapolsky 1990). In marked contrast, the United States, after an initial threat to the blood supply during the first years of the epidemic, has significantly improved the overall quality of its blood services.

Contamination of the blood supply in the United States was first discovered in mid-1982, when three cases of AIDS were found among hemophiliacs. By 1983, blood donors began to be screened, but since the AIDS antibody test was as yet not available, the exclusion of individuals who might be infected was done simply by questionnaires and interviews. Hemophiliacs depend on blood plasma for the clotting factors essential to counteract bleeding. Clotting factors, Sapolsky explains, are derived from pooled plasma lots that are composed of as many as 5,000 donations which can be contaminated by a single AIDS virus carrier. As a consequence, "nearly half of the 15,000 hemophiliacs in the United States are now infected" (289). Screening the volunteers who donate blood and using a heat treatment for plasma have largely removed this danger. However, Sapolsky maintains, because the United States has been the major international supplier of plasma products, the contamination has spread worldwide.

In a review of the prevalence of blood contamination, Miller et al. (1990) refer to a continuing, although minor, problem of contamination despite the universal use of blood testing procedures. Because of the amount of time that elapses between infection by the virus and the development of a detectable antibody response—usually a period of no more than a few months—the blood collected from an infected donor during this "window" period may test negative and remain undetected by the serologic screening techniques of most blood banks.

Blood banks have developed questionnaires concerning risk behavior designed to help potential donors to exclude themselves from donating blood; the questions include a request for a confidential health history. The majority of donors found to be infected had not excluded themselves because they did not believe they were at risk of being infected. In a 1988 survey of donors from urban areas, for example, more than half of infected volunteer donors were in fact bisexuals. A lack of perception of risk has been reported in other studies as well. Estimates of the danger to the blood supply have varied from a rate of one infection for every 40 to 50,000 units transfused to one in every 153,000 units transfused (Miller et al. 1990:291–292). By December 1991, a total of 6,512 cases of AIDS were reported as having been caused by the receipt of blood and blood products (Slutsker et al. 1992:606).

Efforts to dissuade intravenous drug users (IVDUs) from donating or selling blood have not been fully successful. A longitudinal study of 915 intravenous drug users in southern Florida concluded that in spite of these efforts some continue to sell their blood (Chitwood et al. 1991).

The fear of AIDS contamination has had a marked effect on the practice of medicine in the United States. As an illustration, the number of blood transfusions is declining from its all-time high in the early 1980s. It is no longer common, says Sapolsky (1990:293), for a physician to order a unit of blood merely "to put the blush back into the cheeks of a patient about to be discharged from the hospital." And, when considering surgery, physicians and patients alike think harder about the risks of transfusion. As the AIDS epidemic intensifies, the problem is to recruit a "safe" donor—a problem that parallels the one of providing an adequate supply of blood in all blood groups. Increasingly, patients who are able to do so bank their own blood before elective surgery.[11]

The Impact of AIDS on the Health Care System

The AIDS epidemics are having an enormous impact on the health care system in both sub-Saharan Africa and the United States. In Africa, it is pervasive, whereas in the United States, it is selective. In some African countries, the burden of caring for the influx of sick people with the new disease threatens the entire system. The United States—rich, for the most part healthy, equipped with material resources at the cutting edge of technology, and with one of the highest physician–patient ratios in the world—is amply equipped to deal with such an emergency. Yet in the United States AIDS, more than any other single health crisis, has had profound impacts on aspects of the health care system. It has had a transforming effect on the medical profession and has revealed the inadequacies of the entire system of providing adequate and equitable health care for all members of American society.

Impact on the medical profession

The impact of AIDS on the medical profession has been both subtle and increasingly pervasive. Leaders of the profession often comment on the possibility that the epidemic has had a "chilling effect" on the professional culture of physicians in the United States. The most obvious effect has been the mounting pressure on medical personnel in urban academic medical centers where large numbers of AIDS patients are treated. A new cadre of "plague doctors" has arisen to treat patients in public and voluntary hospitals. But as the number of patients has increased, so has the danger of resignations and "burnouts." The emotional, psychological, and physical toll on AIDS professionals is expected to increase as the epidemic grows (Bosk & Frader 1991; Cameron 1992). As the number of persons with HIV/AIDS rises, doctors both in primary health care and in specialties are increasingly being called on to deal with the problems of patients who are often poor, always incurable, and (in some cases) potentially dangerous.

---

[11] For discussions of the implications of the AIDS epidemic for the system of blood services, see Murray (1991) and Sapolsky and Boswell (1992).

The advent of AIDS has thus presented the medical profession with an array of new challenges and ethical dilemmas. It has confronted physicians with a deadly new disease fraught with socially complex problems. During the AIDS era a new sense of personal vulnerability concerning the risk of infection—a feeling that had largely disappeared since the advent of antibiotics—has come into conflict with established norms of professional duty (Schwarz 1989). A major public health threat to increasing numbers of disadvantaged individuals and persons with unconventional life styles, AIDS has created a tension between personal preferences and professional obligations, a tension that David E. Rogers and Eli Ginzburg (1989)—editors of a book on physicians' attitudes toward AIDS patients—term "a national dilemma." There is evidence that a substantial portion of physicians avoid caring for patients with HIV/AIDS. This avoidance or refusal, in addition to denying needed care, stigmatizes patients, and at the same time it increases the risk of infection for those physicians who are willing to treat patients and thus must shoulder a disproportionate burden of the epidemic (Jonsen & Stryker 1993:12).

Contentious issues concerning the right of HIV-infected physicians to continue with their practice have stirred feelings of professional vulnerability. Thus, for Shapiro and his associates (1992:514), authors of a report on Canadian, French, and U.S. physicians' reactions to the pandemic, "the emergence of AIDS is a milestone of sorts for medicine."

The role played by fear. According to Charles Bosk, a medical sociologist, and Joel E. Frader, a physician and an ethicist (who have studied the effects of the emergence of AIDS on the training of physicians in urban teaching centers), the impact of AIDS on medical education has been severe (1991). They cite instances of medical students refusing to deal with AIDS patients, some going so far as to claim that doctors, like lawyers, should have the right to refuse clients. Despite evidence presented in the medical literature that AIDS is not unduly infectious, they report that many doctors are afraid they will become infected. The authors claim that AIDS has eroded the sense of invulnerability so necessary for giving peace of mind to physicians in training. They surmise that among young doctors choosing a career in primary care, fear of AIDS may be aggravating a shift away from such specialties as internal medicine, family practice, and pediatrics to other, more technically oriented specialties.

Ness et al. (1989) report a trend among medical school graduates toward avoiding residencies requiring contact with AIDS patients, particularly pediatrics. The epidemic may have shifted the balance for many neophyte physicians who might have tolerated or even welcomed an opportunity to perform a social service to the financially underprivileged or medically underserved. The effect of these individual decisions, they believe, is that AIDS will bring about a decline in the availability and quality of care for America's underclass served by urban teaching centers. In fact the Ness study of medical students' residency selections during the first decade of the AIDS epidemic showed a trend toward avoidance of residencies in large urban centers with high concentrations of AIDS patients.

Clarke and Conley (1991), in an editorial in the *Journal of the American Medical Association*, call attention to the fact that the rates for filling vacancies in residency programs in urban areas with low incidence of AIDS have remained unchanged, while the "fill rates" for New York City voluntary programs have declined significantly, including voluntary programs in areas of low AIDS incidence. They suspect that medical students may not have bothered to distinguish between high- and low- incidence AIDS programs but simply chose to avoid New York City entirely because of its well-publicized high prevalence of AIDS.

During the first decade of the epidemic, the media reported numerous instances of physicians refusing to treat people infected with HIV. In 1987, Surgeon General C. Everett Koop excoriated this response, saying that it "threatens the very fabric of health care in this country . . . where everyone will be cared for and no one will be turned away" (quoted in Gerbert et al. 1991b:2838).

Increasingly, AIDS is being described by physicians as an occupational disease (Gostin 1989). But fear of becoming infected is a recent phenomenon; in the first years of the epidemic, the possibility of infection was thought to be negligible. By the end of the first decade, however, reports of HIV infection among health care personnel—mostly by hypodermic needle sticks or by splashes of blood from seropositive patients—heightened awareness of HIV as an occupational disease (Brennan 1990). For residents and interns dealing with trauma cases in hospital emergency rooms, the perceived danger is particularly immediate. For surgeons, obstetricians, and dentists who are involved in invasive procedures, AIDS has been increasingly viewed in this way as well (Bell 1990). As Gostin has pointed out, these physicians have claimed the right to know the HIV/AIDS status of their patients; consequently, some hospitals screen patients even without their specific consent.

The continuing interest of medical educators and other leaders of the profession in these issues has sparked a number of attitude surveys—conducted primarily by physicians—among residents, general practitioners, specialists, and other medical care workers. The surveys are designed to determine how a new generation of medical practitioners reacts both to the disease itself and to the threat of infection, how it perceives AIDS patients, and how it actually behaves in the course of medical practice. Some of these surveys seek to obtain such information as the extent to which they have had contact with AIDS patients; the extent of their fear of acquiring AIDS through contact with patients; their recognition of the ethical responsibilities of physicians to provide treatment; and their self-reported attitudes and behavior toward AIDS patients. The studies reviewed and briefly reported upon here are

- The Bresolin et al. (1990) study of 1,500 physicians drawn from the American Medical Association's membership file
- The Colombotos et al. (1991) study of 958 physicians and 1,520 registered nurses
- The Gerbert et al. (1991b) study of 2,004 general internists, family physicians, and general practitioners
- The Rizzo et al. (1990) study of 3,506 physicians, excluding federally employed physicians and residents

The four studies were undertaken for somewhat different purposes; different samples were drawn; and the reports stress different aspects of the relationship of the U.S. medical profession to AIDS. Nonetheless, the studies reached a general consensus on the following:

- There is widespread concern among physicians over becoming HIV-infected through contact with patients. In most studies, more than half of the physicians reported they were concerned or very concerned about this problem.
- The more direct, personal experience physicians have had with AIDS patients, the lower their level of concern.
- A majority of those asked about the obligations of physicians reported their belief that a physician may not ethically refuse to treat a seropositive patient.
- Concern over personal safety does not seem to be a

major reason for leaving or considering leaving
direct patient care.
- The most overarching finding is a conflict in the
  minds of physicians between the obligation to treat
  patients and the fear of contracting AIDS from them.
- Referral seems to be a major method for resolving
  this conflict. For example, in the Colombotos study,
  half of the surgeons said they would not operate on
  a seropositive patient, but none said they would
  refuse to see him. Rather, they would refer him.

Attitudes toward stigmatized groups. A common concern revealed in both the Gerbert and the Colombotos surveys is the degree
to which health care workers are influenced by prevailing attitudes
toward stigmatized groups. Surgeons, obstetricians, hospital
emergency personnel, and dentists are particularly concerned
about their repeated exposure to the blood of HIV-infected patients
(Bell 1990).

In the Gerbert study, over one-third of the physicians expressed
moral disapproval of homosexuals, negative feelings about dealing
with intravenous drug users, antipathy toward vagrants, and
discomfort in dealing with dying AIDS patients. Physicians who had
treated relatively more HIV-infected patients were less negative
toward stigmatized groups: they were less homophobic and expressed
less bias toward drug users. They also reported more professional
gratification and less apprehension about the risk of contagion.

The Colombotos study revealed similar expressions of
prejudice. Both physicians and nurses expressed a reluctance to
care for HIV-infected patients, homosexuals, and intravenous drug
users, nearly two-thirds indicating that they would rather not care
for patients who are HIV positive.

No more than half were "completely willing" to care for
homosexual men and drug users, regardless of their HIV status. In
contrast, 80 percent were willing to care for elderly, black, or
Hispanic patients. Asked whether they would prefer to treat homosexuals with AIDS or drug users with AIDS, only a small percentage
preferred the drug users. In short, the AIDS epidemic has increased
negative feelings toward drug users but not toward male homosexuals.[12]

---

[12] In a summary of physicians' attitudes, M. Roy Schwartz (1989), an official
of the American Medical Association, notes that, as experience in treating
AIDS cases increases, so does tolerance of different life-styles.

A cross-national study of physicians in Canada, France, and the United States (Shapiro et al. (1992) provides insights into how cultural differences influence the treatment of AIDS patients. The physicians studied were either residents in their last year of internal medicine or family medicine residents about to enter medical practice. Most had provided both inpatient and outpatient treatment to AIDS patients in teaching hospitals affiliated with medical schools. Physicians in all three countries expressed a significant fear of contracting AIDS. Although the American residents were more likely than the others to have cared for inpatients with AIDS, needle stick injuries were not uncommon everywhere.

Most of the residents in all three countries viewed their experiences in caring for HIV-infected patients as a positive educational experience, but at the same time many stated that they would prefer not to take care of persons with AIDS or from groups at increased risk of AIDS. The fear of contracting AIDS was significant in all three countries, but it was somewhat less in Canada and France than in the United States, where, of course, there are more HIV-infected patients. Slightly more than one-third of the residents in each country strongly supported the principle that surgeons have a right to know a patient's HIV status before operating.

Despite the latent apprehension brought about by AIDS, a majority of the residents in all three countries were unequivocal in their affirmation of the physician's professional obligation to provide AIDS patients with care. However, given a choice, many residents would prefer not to do so. The reasons expressed reveal a striking difference among the residents in the three countries. The French were less likely to wish to avoid dealing with homosexual men, with AIDS patients, and with intravenous drug users; the American physicians were the least likely to feel an obligation to treat patients without regard for sexual orientation or HIV status; the. Canadian physicians were more likely than the French to stress the ethical need to treat AIDS patients; and the French physicians were more likely to feel that discrimination based on sexual orientation is unethical.[13]

HIV-infected physicians. The beginning of the second decade of AIDS has been marked by increasing controversy concerning the problem of HIV-infected physicians and other health care workers (HCWs). Widespread concern among the U.S public over contracting

---

[13] For a discussion of prejudiced attitudes toward AIDS among the public, see Blendon and Donelan (1989).

HIV from a physician in the course of routine medical care has been documented in a number of surveys. This concern has been matched by a parallel concern among health care workers—particularly by gay and/or HIV-infected physicians and other health care personnel—that their rights and their livelihood could be affected by restrictions placed upon their practice.

Gerbert et al. (1989), in a report on an attitude survey of 2,000 Americans, found that more than half of the respondents said they would change their physician if they learned that the physician was infected. In addition, a quarter would do so if they learned that he or she was treating AIDS patients.

The proposition that a patient who is undergoing seriously invasive surgery has a "right to know" whether or not a physician is HIV positive was buttressed by a 1991 policy statement of the American Medical Association (AMA). The statement revised a 1989 statement that "physicians who are HIV seropositive have an ethical obligation not to engage in any professional activity which has an identifiable risk of transmission of the infection to the patient" (American Medical Association 1991:1). A few months later the American Academy of Orthopaedic Surgeons (AAOS) issued an advisory statement stipulating that "an HIV-infected orthopaedic surgeon should not perform invasive surgical procedures except in the specific, limited instances outlined in the full text of this Advisory Statement" (American Academy of Orthopaedic Surgeons 1991:1).

A cluster of six HIV infections occurring in the patients of a Florida dentist (David J. Acer) in 1990 and the eventual death of one of them (Kimberly Bergalis) accentuated public fears and focused media attention, and ultimately congressional attention as well, on the problem of acquiring AIDS from medical personnel. In response to the Kimberly Bergalis case, in July 1991 the CDC issued guidelines that recommended that health care workers who perform "exposure-prone" invasive procedures should get themselves tested for HIV (and hepatitis B virus) and, if infected, should not perform the procedure without explicit approval from local professional review panels. It also recommended informing patients of the physician's infection (*AIDS Alert*, October 1992:155). This proposal and other more draconian measures proposed by the Senate (including a bill introduced by Senator Jesse Helms of North Carolina to impose criminal penalties of up to a fine of $10,000 and ten years imprisonment for health workers who failed to tell patients of their infection) raised a storm of protest. Most of the forty medical, dental, nursing, and other professional associations refused to cooperate, saying that the guidelines were misleading. The crux of the argument was that the six cases of infection among the patients of the infected dentist were idiosyncratic and that there was little or no evidence to prove dentist-to-patient transmission. Hospital officials, however, interpreting the Senate vote as an expression of growing public fear that health professionals could indeed infect patients, were in favor of cooperating with the guidelines, fearing malpractice suits.

The professional associations' widespread criticism of the CDC guidelines led to their outright rejection by state health departments. New York State, for example, reaffirmed the state's commitment to protect the confidentiality of infected health personnel and allowed them to continue working in most cases (AIDS Alert, January 1992:6). A report by the Office of Technology Assessment of the Congress (Miike et al. 1991) stated that studies by the CDC of more than 4,000 patients of HIV-infected health care workers (so-called look-back studies) had not found any instances of physician-to-patient infection. Even if much larger numbers of patients were to be evaluated, it stated, this method is unlikely to help determine the magnitude of the risk.

The defiance of the CDC guidelines by professional associations led to an amended recommendation on July 18, 1992. The amendment left it up to state health departments to decide, on a case-by-case basis, the type of care that infected physicians and other health care personnel could provide. For advocacy groups such as Physicians for Health Care and the Medical Expertise Retention Program, which represent gay physicians and health care workers, the forced disclosure of HIV status is an unwarranted violation of civil rights and a threat to their livelihood as well.

Lawrence Gostin (1989) examined the issue of a patient's and a physician's right to know about each other and concluded that the physician's right to know that a patient is infected is of limited use because physicians have a professional, if not a legal, responsibility to treat patients regardless. Moreover, the courts have required physicians to give their patients who are faced with seriously invasive surgery all the information they would deem relevant to the decision. The increasing focus of modern law on patients' rights requires a physician to withdraw from performing seriously invasive procedures if a significant risk of HIV infection exists. Gostin believes that there are limits to what society can reasonably expect of a physician in disclosing remote risks.

The gay physicians' advocacy groups advance two main arguments against the mandatory testing of physicians and other health care personnel. First, forced disclosure is unreasonable because the risks of transmission of HIV infection to a patient are remote. However, the gay advocacy argument that the risk of transmission is remote must be set alongside their own estimates of the number of infected health care workers. According to Jonsen and Stryker (1993:61), however, less than 5 percent of all AIDS cases in the United States are known to have been among health care workers (a category that includes physicians and many others). Most, they report, became infected through unprotected sex or intravenous drug use.

Second, the gay physicians advocacy groups argue that physicians, dentists, and nurses are being unfairly targeted by emotional stress lawsuits initiated by uninfected patients against hospital malpractice insurers and health plans for failing to exclude HIV-positive doctors and dentists. These lawsuits increase the incentives for employment discrimination against seropositive professionals (*PAACNOTES*, March/April 1991; Schatz 1991).

In July 1992, the National Commission on AIDS (1992a) issued a report that opposed the CDC guidelines, stating that proposals to restrict the practices of HIV-infected health care workers on the basis of HIV status alone or to inform patients concerning this status are not warranted by the risk of infection and could be counterproductive. In the preface to the report, June E. Osborn and David E. Rogers, chair and vice chair of the Commission, voiced the fear that policies responding to public anxiety concerning HIV transmission in health care settings might result in diminishing, rather than enhancing, public safety and access to quality health care (quoted in *AIDS Alert*, October 1992:154).[14]

Impact on public hospitals

In both sub-Saharan Africa and the United States, a core problem is that of providing both primary services and long-term care for persons with AIDS symptoms. Hospitals are the first line of defense. In the United States, the problem concerns the distribution

---

[14] For another discussion of the problem of HIV infection in the health care setting, see Bell (1990). The sources for the sequence of events concerning HIV-infected physicians are the following 1991 issues of the *New York Times*: June 16:C7; July 19:A1, A14; July 20:13; August 20:C1, C5; August 30:A1, A19; October 4:18; October 9:A1, B6; and October 15:C3.

of health care, not the lack of medical resources. In the first decade of the epidemic, the public hospital system responded to the crisis by changing the conventions for patient treatment, establishing special inpatient and outpatient clinics for AIDS patients, and dedicating entire institutions as centers for treatment (Lloyd 1988). However, the increase in the number of HIV and AIDS cases, particularly in areas of high incidence in large and medium-sized urban centers, is taxing the resources of public hospitals in these areas, already burdened as they are with dealing with thousands of low- income or indigent patients for whom the emergency room is a substitute for the family physician (Drucker 1991:61).[15]

As the National Commission on AIDS noted in its report *America Living with AIDS* (1991c), the expected increase in the number of HIV and AIDS cases will be the final straw for a system that is already on the verge of collapse. As prophylaxis and treatment for opportunistic infections improve and even larger numbers of patients seek antiviral therapy as new drugs become available, the number of persons living with HIV and AIDS will increase. In addition, people infected with HIV who have severe immunosuppression without AIDS-defining illness would also require care, creating an urgent demand for new resources (Slutsker et al. 1992).[16] Abandoned children who are HIV-infected and drug-exposed are part of a broader abandoned baby problem that plagues inner-city hospitals (National Commission on AIDS 1992b).

The seriousness of the imminent threat to the nation's medical care system was stated dramatically by June Osborn in the course of an interview (*New York Times*, November 2, 1992:B10). "People are literally dying in the streets," she reported. "This is going to get very, very big. It seems big now, but you ain't seen nothing yet."

A report on health care services in eleven cities throughout the country, funded by the Robert Wood Johnson Foundation (Weisfeld 1991), assesses the impact of AIDS on the entire system and comes to a pessimistic conclusion:

- AIDS has challenged the system to a greater degree

---

[15] In inner-city communities in New York City, understaffed and underfunded municipal hospitals serve areas where HIV/AIDS is concentrated and health insurance is lacking. Thirteen of the 72 New York hospitals serve over half of the city's AIDS patients (Jonsen & Stryker 1993:271).

[16] For an extended analysis of the impact of AIDS on the health care system, see Strauss et al. (1991); for analyses of its specific impact on the hospital system, see Killip (1989) and Levine (1990a).

any other single medical condition.

- This is so because of the nature of the illness, which requires frequent hospital stays, access to outpatient as well as inpatient services, and help in coping with the tasks of daily living as patients deteriorate. In short, care for AIDS parallels the needs of the elderly and the chronically ill.
- The demands of AIDS, combined with the demands resulting from drug use, have stretched the health care system of large cities beyond endurance; public hospitals are "on the brink of collapse."
- The treatment demands of the HIV-infected, seeking to delay the onset of symptoms with new therapeutic drugs and other therapies, will cause additional strain on an already faltering system.

The expected impact of advanced AIDS disease in diagnostic and treatment centers will be especially dramatic because of the presence of dementia which affects patients in the last stages. Justin C. McArthur (1992), a neurologist at the Johns Hopkins University, writes that assuming 400,000 cumulative AIDS cases by the end of 1993, of which 30 percent develop dementia, there will be about 120,000 individuals with HIV dementia. (In contrast, Alzheimer's disease develops in about 150,000 Americans annually.) HIV/AIDS may add approximately 30,000 more cases of dementia each year, requiring diagnostic tests and care that, although short-term, is very intensive.

The very nature of AIDS creates organizational problems for hospitals. Although many AIDS sufferers wish to end their days at home, they end up dying in hospitals because of the inadequacies of home care services (Strauss et al. 1991). The need for hospital beds fluctuates: the problem of planning for in-patient hospital beds is one example. As more therapies for treating the multiplicity of symptoms that characterize HIV infection are developed, fewer persons will need to be hospitalized.

Another example of the evolution of AIDS care which compounds the organizational problems of hospitals is the fact that HIV disease attacks every organ system of the body. The U.S. health care system has been criticized in the past for not providing comprehensive and coordinated primary care and for relying too much on specialties and subspecialties. Yet AIDS demands the primary care that is necessary to cope with a disabling disease "that stubbornly refuses to be limited to any single organ system" (Jonsen & Stryker

1993:49).

Jonsen and Stryker (51–53) also emphasize that AIDS has prompted a reexamination of the philosophy underlying hospital care. The experience of dealing with the episodic nature of the disease, and its evolution into being a chronic rather than solely a terminal illness, have led to this reevaluation. With some nursing homes refusing to accept AIDS patients, specialized hospice care facilities have been established for patients in the terminal stage. Jonsen and Stryker point out that hospice health care is now a billion dollar a year business (68).

The Economic Impact of AIDS

The costs of AIDS

The AIDS crisis saddles public hospitals with new financial burdens with each municipal budget. The fundamental problem according to Armstrong and Bos (1992) is the lack of universal care coverage, which means that an increasing share of the costs of AIDS care is being assumed by public sector health facilities that are not reimbursed fully by Medicaid/Medicare programs.

A survey of hospitals (*New York Times*, May 13, 1992:A17) examined the admissions of HIV-infected individuals who were not classified as AIDS patients in 325 private and public hospitals and concluded that current estimates severely underreport the needs and costs of such patients. (The study was the first to examine the costs of HIV care and not just of AIDS patients with classic recognized symptoms.) In an interview at the time the study report was released, Lawrence M. Barat, an adviser on AIDS policy to the city of Boston, declared that these findings constituted further evidence that the CDC should broaden the definition of AIDS to include more symptoms.[17] Most of the HIV-patients in the study were uninsured members of inner-city minorities who had become infected through contaminated drug injections. Public hospitals bear the financial burden of treating such patients, but since they are supported by tax dollars, they are being forced to shoulder a

---

[17] A broadened definition was adopted on January 1, 1993, to assist health officials gauge the extent of the epidemic. The new definition will help capture many cases among women and drug users who had been left out under the old definition. It is expected to nearly double the number of new AIDS cases reported nationwide (*New York Times*, January 6, 1993:B3).

disproportionate share of the burden of caring for patients with only publicly financed coverage or no coverage at all, according to Bartlett (1990:213). Both public and private hospitals cover their losses on uninsured patients either by increasing their charges to patients who can pay for their care or by increasing their revenues from taxes. This, says Bartlett, "can be viewed as a hidden tax that society ultimately pays in the form of higher charges or higher taxes" (213). Health economists Bloom and Carliner (1988) make a similar point, stressing that private hospitals, because they cannot operate indefinitely with ever larger losses from AIDS patients, have simply increased the charges made to patients who are covered by insurance.

Estimates of what AIDS costs the U. S. health system and the entire U.S. economy varied widely during the first decade of the epidemic. It could hardly have been otherwise, since the definition of who is afflicted with AIDS has changed and the definition of what costs should be included as AIDS costs have not been uniform. But as the contours of the epidemic emerged more clearly and as more HIV-infected individuals and AIDS patients sought treatment, a general consensus on these costs began to emerge during the early 1990s.

Fred J. Hellinger (1991), a health economist with the U.S. Department of Health and Human Services, reported in a pioneering article that AIDS cost the U.S. economy $5.8 billion in 1991, an annual outlay that is expected to increase to $10 billion by 1994. Nevertheless, the costs of AIDS are said to constitute only 1 percent of total health care costs in the United States (Armstrong & Bos 1992). Although 1 percent of national health care costs seems minor, the financing of care for the uninsured poor is becoming a burden for local governments that depend on federal Medicaid funds. The local financial burden in high-incidence areas is substantial; furthermore, Medicaid is facing cutbacks in many states (Jonsen & Stryker 1993:68).

The annual cost of treating an individual infected with HIV but who has not yet developed AIDS is estimated to be $5,150; the estimated annual cost for an AIDS patient is $32,000; and the lifetime cost is calculated to be $85,333. Earlier figures, Hellinger reported, underestimated the costs of medical care because they were limited to the treatment of full-blown AIDS. The advent of new drugs to delay the onset of the disease (25 percent of all HIV-patients receive them), as well as the fact that AIDS patients are living longer, has significantly increased the costs of dealing with AIDS. One year later, however, these costs had escalated further. Reporting to the 1992 international AIDS conference in Amsterdam, Hellinger said that the annual treatment cost for an AIDS patient in the United States was then $38,300; for an HIV-infected individual, the cost had almost doubled to $10,000. The lifetime costs of treating an AIDS patient has now escalated to $102,000 (*New York Times*, July 23, 1992).

Bruce C. Vladeck (1989), president of the United Hospital Fund of New York, characterized the financial plight of people with the AIDS virus in stark terms. He noted that most people with AIDS are poor, and if they are not poor to begin with, they soon become poor as they lose their jobs and pay their medical bills. The reason for this state of affairs, as *America Living with AIDS* (National Commission on AIDS 1991c) reports, is that the linking of private insurance to employment is problematic for people with AIDS. Consequently, many AIDS patients with limited resources (mainly poor blacks and Hispanics) turn to Medicaid, the federal insurance program for the indigent. Medicaid has become the most important source of financing for AIDS. It covers 40 per cent of all adults and 90 per cent of all children with AIDS. This situation has been dubbed the "Medicaidization" of AIDS, which is defined as a shift in the distribution of individuals with third-party financing from private insurance to Medicaid (Green & Arno 1990). In an analysis of the task of financing health care for persons with AIDS, Lawrence Bartlett (1990), a health systems analyst, has pointed out that the epidemic has generated fear in addition to the fear of contracting AIDS. Specifically, employers and employees fear for the impact of AIDS on their health costs; managers of public health care programs fear for the impact on their budgets; public hospitals fear for their financial viability; and HIV-infected persons fear for their health benefits (as well as for their lives, of course). Bartlett points out, however, that AIDS patients are not alone in falling through the gaps in the U.S. health care system; an estimated 37 million people have no health care insurance at all and may risk facing financial ruin if they acquire a serious illness.

The National Commission on AIDS has eloquently described the role of AIDS in worsening the problems of medical care in the United States:

> The HIV epidemic did not leave 37 million or more Americans without ways to finance their medical care . . . but it did dramatize their plight. The HIV epidemic did not cause the problem of homelessness —but it has

expanded it and made it more visible. The HIV epidemic did not cause the collapse of the health care system— but it has accelerated the disintegration of our hospitals and intensified their problems. The HIV epidemic did not directly augment problems of substance abuse but it has made the need for drug treatment for all who require it a matter of urgent national priority. Rural health care, prison health care, access to health care for uninsured and underinsured working men and women—these issues and many more form the fabric of our concern (National Commission on AIDS 1991c:4).

Jonsen and Stryker (1993) confirm the aggravating rather than the causative role of AIDS. The epidemic has expanded the "fissures" already present in the medical insurance system, they affirm. It has compounded demands—from both health care providers struggling to cope with uninsured patients and patients struggling to pay for drugs and services. Thus, they point out, "another voice has been added to the call for a comprehensive solution to the problem of health care financing" (13).

Lost economic potential

As in the case of Africa, although on a much smaller scale, the loss of human economic potential is one of the important but hidden consequences of the AIDS epidemic. The National Commission pointed out in its 1991 report that health economists calculate this cost in terms of "years of potential life lost"[18]—a summation of the years of economic productivity lost between age 65 and death. Because AIDS is a disease of the young, who generally die in the first half of their careers, each death from AIDS contributes more to this cost than does a life lost from cancer, heart disease, or stroke, which are primarily but, of course, not entirely diseases of older people. The years of life lost from these diseases remain stable from year to year, while the lost years resulting from AIDS continue to rise. In 1991, AIDS ranked third among all diseases in this calculus, behind cancer and heart disease, and "by 1993 AIDS will clearly outstrip all other diseases in lost human potential" (National Commission on

---

[18] One year of "potential life lost" is defined as the year between the actual death of a person and the year in which he or she would have reached age 65. See National Commission on AIDS (1991c:13).

AIDS 1991c:13).

    There are other measures of lost economic potential. In 1992, federal expenses for AIDS totaled $5 billion; nonfederal payments for treatment totaled $8 billion; and the future loss in federal and state tax revenue because of deaths from AIDS in 1992 was expected to total $15 billion to $20 billion (*New York Times*, November 22, 1992:111-11). Undoubtedly there are other significant costs not included in this summary of two brief computations.

Loss of manpower in the arts

    Unlike other major causes of death such as cancer and heart disease, AIDS primarily affects people in the labor force. For this reason, the potential loss of manpower is an integral aspect of the difficult calculus for determining socioeconomic costs. In sub-Saharan Africa, the loss of educated and talented government officials, professionals, and businessmen is threatening the viability of some countries. In the United States, there is no evidence of such an impact upon the comparable elites, but the high mortality rate among male homosexuals is having a devastating effect on the arts.

    Hardly a day goes by without the appearance of an obituary—in the major newspapers of New York, San Francisco, and Los Angeles, particularly—announcing the death from AIDS of one or more young or middle-aged professionals in some field of the arts: architecture, dance, film, music, painting, television, the theater, writing, and so on, or in such trades as fashion design, interior decorating, or the sale of antiques. Some 200–300 such obituaries appear annually in the *New York Times*—and of course the deaths of only the most prominent of these people are recorded in its pages.

    Richard Goldstein (1991:17), arts editor of the *Village Voice* in New York City, noted that when AIDS first appeared few cultural critics foresaw the epidemic's impact on the arts. "But ten years later," he said, "it is possible to argue that virtually every form of art or entertainment in America has been touched by AIDS." The death from AIDS of the ballet dancer Rudolf Nureyev in 1993 led to a large number of press stories about the problem (e.g., "A Lost Generation":1993).

    The loss of thousands of talented people engaged in one aspect of American cultural life is, of course, a loss to the nation's talent pool. But the obituaries show another, more subtle effect, on the culture. They increasingly follow a common pattern: AIDS is explicitly given as the cause of death, even when the more proximate cause is known, and the deceased's companion is often mentioned as the principal survivor.

AIDS and the Future of Medical Care

Observers of the AIDS epidemic in the United States believe it has profound implications for the future of the national health care system. In the second decade of the epidemic, HIV/AIDS has come to be increasingly perceived by public health officials and the medical profession as requiring a response akin to other lethal chronic diseases such as cancer, heart disease, and stroke—all of which require specialized long-term care that prolongs life but generally does not provide a cure (Fee & Fox 1992, Introduction; Fox 1992). This conclusion has important implications for the future of health care in the United States. The medical sociologist Anselm L. Strauss and his colleagues (1991) posit that by exacerbating the drain on medical resources, the AIDS epidemic has thrown into sharp relief the dilemmas of choice, the differences within, and the fundamental inequities of the entire system of providing care for Americans. Specifically:

- AIDS has intensified the moral and ethical issues involved in ongoing dilemmas of choice. It has added a new dimension to the problem of balancing the competing needs of the larger public against those of the terminally ill, of the elderly, of "worst case" infants not allowed to die, and of premature infants with long-term expensive disabilities.
- AIDS has raised the old issue of personal responsibility for illness, which Strauss and his colleagues describe as "an absurd and ethically dishonest concept to apply to economically deprived Americans" (64). Indeed, they report, AIDS may turn out to be the experimental ground for managing illness among the homeless (70).
- AIDS has highlighted the organizational difficulties of a system geared to acute care rather than the care of chronic illness. Both hospitals and clinics are fundamentally still organized to provide acute care. The system is not organized, for example, to provide home care for sufferers in the last stages of a terminal illness. Hospices are strained to capacity, and the burden of caring for terminally ill patients has fallen on voluntary gay community groups. It can be anticipated that, as the ranks of those sick with AIDS swell and overwhelm hospitals and clin-

ics, the health care system will be forced to incorpo-
rate more home care services.

- Because of the AIDS experience, the present system
  of "high-tech" acute care medicine will be reas-
  sessed and redesigned in the light of the prevalence
  of chronic illnesses of all kinds.
- The current system, aggravated by the burden of the
  AIDS epidemic, implies a rationing of care. The
  economic implication is that Americans will have to
  rethink what portion of the GNP they wish to assign
  to health as opposed to many other competing
  claims.

The observation that the advent of AIDS may require a
rationing of patient care in the United States finds support in the
warning of historians Elizabeth Fee and Daniel M. Fox (1992:5), who
point out that "today the problem of health policy is not so much to
provoke a more generous official response to AIDS as to make sure
that other health programs are not sacrificed to feed the swelling
budgets appropriated for AIDS research and services." For public
health analyst Ronald Bayer (1991a:95), the dilemmas of choice are
even more stark. Using New York City as an extreme example of what
may eventually occur elsewhere, he suggests that the present
medical care system may force a rationing of resources. He cites the
choices between providing care for AIDS cases and nursing homes
for the aged, between providing care for single adults with AIDS and
apartments for homeless families with children, and between assisting
HIV-infected women and noninfected women who need access to
drug abuse treatment programs. Quoting a phrase of Bruce Vladeck's,
Bayer concludes that making these choices requires a "calculus of
misery."

Assessing the Impacts of AIDS on Social Institutions

The end of the first decade of AIDS has stimulated a burgeoning
literature of individual commentary seeking to evaluate selected
aspects of the U.S. epidemic. Predictably, the prime focus has
been—as indicated earlier in this chapter—on the impact of a new
epidemic disease on the health care system, since this involves the
key institutions most directly affected. But these overt manifestations of impact tend to obscure a host of more subtle transforma-
tions that are occurring in other segments of American society. In
the second decade of AIDS, these pervasive sociocultural changes—

positive as well as negative—are becoming more apparent and are increasingly the subject of analysis by observers of the epidemic from a wide range of disciplines.

In 1989, the National Research Council, which serves as the research arm of the National Academy of Sciences, appointed a Committee on AIDS Research and the Social, Behavioral, and Statistical Sciences for the purpose of studying aspects of the AIDS epidemic and making recommendations to the government. The committee has issued three reports: Turner et al., *AIDS: Sexual Behavior and Intravenous Drug Use* (1989), and Miller et al., *AIDS: The Second Decade* (1990) are referred to in Chapter 7. The third report is Jonsen and Stryker, *The Social Impact of AIDS* (1993).[19] The intent of this report, according to the panel of scholars responsible for it, is "to capture and describe" the ways in which selected social institutions have responded to and been transformed by the HIV/AIDS epidemic. The attempt is to identify those changes that will endure or that "must be taken into account in the next decade." Even "partial" or "apparently transitory" responses are seen as indicating a more fundamental change (3).

The report limits its assessments of the social impact of the epidemic to eight areas: (1) public health practice, (2) the role of voluntary associations and community-based organizations, (3) public policies concerning children and families, (4) clinical research and drug regulation, (5) the HIV epidemic in New York City, (6) health care delivery and financing, (7) correctional institutions, and (8) religion and religious groups. In the following summary of its conclusions, only the chapters on the first five topics are reviewed.

Public health practice

The AIDS epidemic has revolutionized the public health management of infectious disease. In response to pressure from well-organized gay community groups and their allies in both medical and political establishments, public health officials have adopted a new approach to the containment of AIDS (41). This "collaborative relationship" has allowed public health officials to

---

[19] The report was edited by the medical ethicist Albert R. Jonsen and the health policy analyst Jeff Stryker, under the auspices of an advisory panel representing anthropology, economics, health policy, history of medicine, law, medical sociology and psychology, and medical and theological ethics. Some of its conclusions have already been noted in this chapter

negotiate with communities that are normally antagonistic to government agencies. Traditional measures such as quarantine, mandatory testing to identify infected individuals, and contact tracing of the partners of infected patients (all of which have notable disadvantages in dealing with a disease having a long latency, which is spread by sexual activity or intravenous drug use, and which is most prevalent among stigmatized groups) were abandoned. They were superseded by community education efforts and voluntary, anonymous testing. These new measures represent an "exceptionalist" policy that differs radically from responses to previous epidemics. The report evaluates the impact of this new approach on the public health system as being "pervasive" (10).

In the second decade of AIDS, however, some aspects of this innovative approach may be superseded by a return to modified versions of the traditional approach because of the availability of early treatments for HIV requiring early identification of infection.

Role of voluntary associations

The AIDS crisis has provided new opportunities for volunteer groups of citizens to participate in the battle against disease. The involvement of volunteers, primarily from the gay community, in hundreds of community-based voluntary associations is "one of the defining characteristics of the epidemic" (173).[20] In the second decade of the epidemic, however, social, cultural, and psychological difficulties resulting from dealing with the marginalized and deprived communities in which the epidemic is spreading may render the contribution of volunteers futile precisely when they are most needed.

Children and families

AIDS has affected the law in the United States in diverse ways, both in legislation and in litigation. The NRC impact-assessment panel, considering its overall impact on the legal system as too diffuse to evaluate, focused on (1) policies affecting newborns and children with HIV disease and (2) the recognition of unmarried couple relationships. Concerning the first topic, the panel emphasized that the epidemic has pushed to extremes "the burdens and

---

[20] For a discussion of the role of nationwide voluntary associations, particularly of the Gay Men's Health Crisis (GMHC) and of ACT-UP, see Kobasa (1991).

responsibilities of caretakers and the state" (203). All children of HIV-infected mothers require special care until they die, a "highly probable" outcome. Pediatric AIDS thus provides an occasion to examine the impact of this "new, chronic, and fatal illness" on infants who are overwhelmingly poor and black or Hispanic. It has highlighted the very question of the allocation of responsibility among parents, extended families, foster parents, and the state. The most important impact of AIDS on social policies concerning AIDS among children has been to force a response by existing social service systems, which are already overburdened, and to show up inconsistencies and anomalies in government policies.

The panel also examined the role AIDS has played in shaping the struggles leading to new housing rules that protect the partners in same-sex relationships in both New York City and San Francisco. Lobbying by gay rights and AIDS organizations in tenant–landlord disputes has been crucial. In a precedent-setting case in New York City, the surviving member of a gay couple, Miguel Braschi, sued successfully in court to remain living in his deceased partner's rent-controlled apartment. The *Braschi* decision expanded the definition of the family to include "two adult life-time partners whose relationship is long-term and characterized by an emotional and financial commitment and interdependence" (quoted in Jonsen & Stryker 1993:234). The panel concluded that AIDS, "a fatal disease, associated in the public mind with promiscuous sexual acts . . . nevertheless contributed to the recognition and acceptance of a variety of emotionally intimate and interdependent family ties that were once outside the law" (238).[21]

Clinical research and drug regulation

AIDS has had its most telling impact on the clinical testing and regulation of new drugs: it has exposed the arena of clinical investigation—the organization, ethics, and politics of research—to media and public scrutiny (80). The result has been a dramatic increase in public awareness of the clinical trials conducted to test new drugs for treatment. Jonsen and Stryker observe that AIDS has both publicized and politicized aspects of clinical investigation that were formerly within the private purview of the scientific community. This process has broad implications for both the conduct of

---

[21] For further discussion of the impact of AIDS on the institution of the family, see Levine (1991).

scientific research and the practice of medicine. In effect, the report underscores that, "to a degree that few would have anticipated, AIDS has influenced the nature and meaning of human experimentation" (112).

The onset of AIDS has created "a constituency of individuals eager to take risks with unproven therapies" (13)—a development that has influenced (if not transformed) the standard process by which new drugs are tested and approved. Randomized clinical trials that assign human subjects to experimental and control groups has been a standard method of clinical investigation. This research tradition, the report points out, has always been fraught with conflicts between the need for scientific knowledge and the welfare of individual participants. (This conflict is sometimes described as "the Arrowsmith dilemma," named for the protagonist of Sinclair Lewis's 1925 novel, a young doctor who had to choose between maintaining the integrity of a controlled experiment and providing medicine for patients in the control group.)

Pressure from AIDS advocates has led to a reevaluation of the traditional double-blind, placebo-controlled clinical trials that have strict entry criteria. AIDS patients and their advocates have pressured successfully for approval of participation by community-based physicians and their patients in "parallel track" trials. The American Foundation for AIDS Research and the National Institute of Allergy and Infectious Diseases responded by establishing a network of community-based trials. In addition, advocates have argued for increased access to trials on a demographically representative basis, including minorities, intravenous drug users, and women. (Women have traditionally been excluded from clinical trials of other diseases despite NIH guidelines requiring their participation.) Thus, the report notes, although AIDS was not the cause of the debate concerning the inclusion of women, it has sharpened the debate because it is now a leading cause of death among women of child-bearing age.[22]

In addition to providing expanded access to clinical trials, AIDS has also stimulated a critical reevaluation of the traditional practices of peer review of submissions to scientific and medical journals, a process that generally delays disclosure of information concerning new research results. In the past decade, authors, journalists, physicians, and public health officials have protested

---

[22] For a comparison of placebo trials in cancer and AIDS research, and their implications, see Rothman and Edgar (1992).

these delays. As a result, some journals have adopted "fast-track" methods of manuscript review, and government agencies have requested permission to release information to the lay press and to practicing physicians prior to its actual publication in journals. The scientific community is grappling with the problem of implementing a "more pragmatic yet still responsible" approach to peer review (14).

The epidemic has also produced another innovation: medical newsletters that disseminate AIDS information to professionals and patients alike.[23] "The dissemination of AIDS research information through AIDS-specific nontraditional means," the report states," has been explosive" (110).   Many mainstream researchers and clinicians are subscribers, even contributors, and these publications effectively fill the gap between peer-reviewed journals and the mass media.

Evaluating the social impact of HIV/AIDS on clinical research and the regulation of new drugs the report noted:

> It is apparent that patient activism, a political climate favoring deregulation, and the exigencies of the AIDS epidemic have generated the most significant reevaluation of the research and regulation processes to occur since World War II . . . . AIDS has led to fundamental reconsideration of basic methodologies for establishing the efficacy and safety of pharmaceuticals. New approaches to experimentation . . . are actively being explored . . . The very legitimacy of randomization has been called into question as the ethics of withholding treatments has loomed large in the context of the epidemic (111–112).

As a consequence, the panel stresses, attempts will probably be made to expedite the regulatory process for drugs for those diseases that are life-threatening. However, reports of drug-related ill effects—toxicity, morbidity, and drug-related mortality—could lead to new restrictions.[24]

---

[23] *AIDS Treatment News* and *PI Perspectives* (published by Project Inform), both published in San Francisco, reach 55,000 readers, including mainstream clinicians and researchers (Jonsen & Stryker 1993:110).

[24] For a different analysis of the problems of drug regulation and human experimentation, and an opposite evaluation of the innovations brought about by the AIDS epidemic. see Edgar and Rothman (1991).

Finally, in this accounting, the report states that "to a degree that few could have anticipated, AIDS has influenced the nature and meaning of the ethics of human investigation" (112). The epidemic has forced science to accelerate the procedures and processes of clinical investigation, as well as the mechanisms of regulation—a process that was beginning prior to AIDS in earlier demands for cancer drugs.

Nevertheless, the research community is seriously concerned that what has been considered an effective research tool may be compromised and that the safety and efficacy of new therapies have not been fully evaluated. Thus, the panel concludes, the long-term impact of these new approaches is not known. These changes must be viewed in the context of the powerful social and political activism generated by the epidemic, typified by the activist slogan "a drug trial is health care too."

The HIV epidemic in New York City

In a study of the epidemic in New York City, which the panel characterizes as an atypical, "highly localized" example, the panel reached the conclusion that the epidemic is exceptional in the sense that it "can only be appreciated when one examines the complex of social and biological problems with which it constantly interacts" (296).

New York City suffers, the report states, from a "synergy of plagues" that emerge in certain areas. The people who inhabit these areas will be devastated far more seriously than the population of the nation at large. These are the inner-city poor, living in "invisible neighborhoods" within the "segregated communities" of the city. The epidemic that has already caused 30,000 deaths and may eventually cause 200,000 will have devastating human consequences, but it "will have passed through the city without fundamental impacts on the life of the city" (296). As in similar areas in cities throughout the country, the social institutions that provide care for the afflicted are already overburdened or nonexistent.

Two overriding conclusions of the report are that (1) the AIDS epidemic, despite having brought devastating sickness and death, has not "significantly altered the structures or directions of the social institutions studied," and that (2) the epidemic has largely impacted socially marginalized groups. Many geographical areas and strata of the U.S. population are virtually untouched by the epidemic and probably never will be, but certain confined areas and populations have been devastated and are likely to continue to be

(7). Within these "socially-separated" marginalized groups, AIDS is becoming endemic but has not spread to the general population.

In an introduction and summary of the report, Jonsen and Stryker disagree with the editors of a book of essays purporting to assess the social impact of the AIDS epidemic in the United States. The book is *A Disease of Society* (Nelkin et al. 1991), whose fundamental premise is that

> More than a passing tragedy, it [AIDS] will have long-term, broad-ranging effects on personal relationships, social institutions, and cultural configurations . . . AIDS will also *reshape* many aspects of society, its institutions, its norms and values, its interpersonal relationships, and its cultural representations . . . The future will be unlike both the present and the past (1–2).

Rejecting this interpretation, the panel concludes that in its ultimate impact the U.S. AIDS epidemic will resemble the flu epidemic of 1918 more than the bubonic plague of 1348. "Many of its most striking features will be absorbed in the flow of American life, but, hidden beneath the surface, its worst effects will continue to devastate the lives and cultures of certain communities"(6).

4

The International
Response

Any assessment of the social consequences of the AIDS pandemic must include its extraordinary impact on international relations. The fear and in some cases the panic engendered by AIDS have triggered two dramatically different reactions. The first has been a negative, defensive reaction expressed by governments and by hostile press and media coverage that threatened to sour international relations—particularly in the first years of the AIDS pandemic. The second, in marked contrast, is an overwhelmingly positive, unprecedented cooperative global effort to combat the epidemic.

Xenophobic reactions to AIDS

More than fifty countries all over the world have imposed exclusionary restrictions on the international travel and immigration of people with HIV and AIDS, ranging from tourism to business travel, to immigration, to student exchanges (Tomasevski 1992:555). Belgium, Bulgaria, Czechoslovakia, Costa Rica, Cuba, France, Hungary, Iraq, Kuwait, Saudi Arabia, South Korea, the former Soviet Union, Sweden, Thailand, the United Arab Emirates, and the United States are among the countries that already employ mandatory testing of blood for all but short-term visitors. Reactions to AIDS in sub-Saharan African countries have been similar to those in Europe and North America—with compulsory screening of both immigrants and entering students (Krisber & Blaney 1987). Algeria, Morocco, and Syria, on the other hand, test the blood of all returning nationals.

The Indian Council of Medical Research has proposed that sex relations with an infected foreigner be made a criminal offense punishable by a fine or a prison sentence. Foreign students cannot enroll in Indian universities without HIV clearance certificates and visitors who want to stay in India for more than three months are subjected to mandatory testing (Misztal & Moss 1990:10). China limits contacts between its citizens and foreigners. In South Africa, migrant workers from neighboring states who are found to be HIV positive are deported. In Japan, which has had relatively few cases but which is experiencing an increase, a prevention campaign poster urges caution while traveling abroad by depicting a man carrying his passport—indicating that the danger is in catching the disease while away from Japan (*New York Times*, November 8, 1992:13).

In the United States, infection with HIV is one of the conditions that can bar entry to immigrants, refugees, and visitors (unless visitors can obtain a waiver). This policy has been fraught with controversy and has been repeatedly criticized by public health experts within the government, as well as by numerous AIDS advocacy organizations, as being needlessly discriminatory. The reality is that some 1 million people in the United States are already infected with HIV. In January 1991, Louis Sullivan, the U.S secretary of health and human services, proposed that aliens with HIV not be excluded from the United States because they would not pose a significant additional risk of HIV infection to the U.S. population, since AIDS cannot be transmitted by casual contact (*New York Times*, January 4, 1991:A1, A15).

Publication of the Sullivan proposal in the *Federal Register* raised a storm of protest in the Congress as well as from conservative groups all over the country. Representative William E. Dannemeyer, Republican of California, attacked the proposal as being inconsistent: "On the one hand they say AIDS is a major problem; on the other hand, they say we should take in AIDS carriers with impunity." Others objected that allowing infected aliens to enter would expose the country to potentially huge medical costs. The issue was debated for the next two years by both the public and the Congress. Finally, on March 11, 1993, the House of Representatives followed an earlier vote in the Senate and voted "to ban immigration into the United States by people infected with the virus that causes AIDS" (*New York Times*, March 12, 1993: A11).[1]

---

[1] For additional details of this controversy, see the later section of this chapter, "The annual AIDS conferences: An international forum."

As in the case of such diseases as syphilis and smallpox, other countries, generally the United States or the countries of sub-Saharan Africa, are often blamed for AIDS. In France, as Dennis Altman (1986) observed, AIDS was at least initially seen as an American import. In the United Kingdom, AIDS has been blamed on homosexuals who have been on sex holidays to America. Dorothy Nelkin and Sander L. Gilman reported that the French labeled AIDS an "American disease" as early as 1981, referring to the American influence on French attitudes toward homosexuality. For some segments of the French public, they noted, "AIDS was but another example of the American corruption of the French body politic, but now in the form of a 'real disease.'" Amyl nitrate "poppers," used to enhance sexual experience during homosexual acts, were labeled "an American pollutant consumed here." The French government warned the gay "jet set" that it was at risk because of the "American connection" (Nelkin & Gilman 1988:364).

In India, consorting with foreigners is the focus of blame. In a lead story in the weekly magazine *Sunday*, A. S. Paintal (1989), director of the Indian Council of Medical Research, declared "AIDS is being poured into women. If women (prostitutes) had taken steps two years ago and stopped cohabiting with foreigners, then the situation would not have become so dangerous." In the Philippines, suspicions that American military personnel were potential carriers of AIDS to the local population became part of the discussions concerning the renewal of American bases and provoked angry polemics in Japan (Ergas 1987).[2]

The "blame the foreigner" syndrome has been most in evidence in the widely reported series of accusatory exchanges that have characterized the reciprocal attitudes of Westerners and Africans and that have had a deleterious impact on foreign relations. As a "classic" instance of Europeans blaming Africans for AIDS, the Panos Dossier (1989:76) cited a sensational article in the British *Sunday Telegraph* (September 21, 1986), which claimed that British diplomats in Tanzania, Uganda, and Zambia had warned that African visitors to Britain could be a primary source of infection and should be subjected to blood screening. Despite the British

---

[2] Ergas called attention to another potentially inhibiting effect on international relations of foreign suspicions of Americans as transmitters of AIDS, that is, the U. S. Department of State announcement in December 1986 that a test for HIV seropositivity would be required of all employees and their dependents stationed overseas.

government's disavowal of any plans to screen Zambians, the Zambian minister of health threatened reciprocation and labeled AIDS a capitalist disease. One damaging result of the exchange was that British physicians and researchers working with Zambian colleagues on AIDS projects were told that the collaboration could not continue. The rash of accusations spread to other African countries and led both to denials of the seriousness of the epidemic and to delays in launching control programs. Nigeria tried to wish it away, as the Nigerian magazine *Newswatch* admitted in March 1987, and thus lost precious time in responding to the crisis.

Aside from seeing the attempts to blame them for the epidemic as a political insult, the African governments have had an economic motivation. African ministers in charge of tourism have been worried about the potentially deleterious effect on tourism, a major source of foreign revenue. Zambians attributed the decline of tourist revenues in 1985 to unfavorable reports in the British press concerning the prevalence of AIDS among Zambian students in Britain. The Kenyan government was particularly upset by erroneous media reports originating in Boston, London, and Stockholm concerning the prevalence of AIDS in Kenya. It expressed its anger at the Western press by confiscating copies of the *International Herald Tribune* that carried a *New York Times* story on AIDS in Kenya (Waite 1989).

The Africans' outraged response to what they perceived as racial stereotyping is eloquently summarized in an article entitled "The Spread of Racism" in the journal *West Africa* (Chirimuuta et al. 1988). The article maintained that the uncontrolled sexuality of black people is a continuing theme of racist mythology used, for example, to justify the lynching of innocent black people in the southern United States. When AIDS first appeared in black people, in the minds of white people it changed almost overnight from a "gay plague" to being an imported Haitian disease and then to being an African disease. Many black people, the authors assert, view the Haitian and African connections with a profound skepticism.

The "blame the foreigner" syndrome found a different expression in the Soviet disinformation campaign (launched in 1985 at the height of the Cold War) directed against the United States. As Nelkin and Gilman (1988:361) report, the AIDS virus was described in articles published in the *Literaturnaya Gazeta*, the official journal of the Soviet Writers Union, as the product of biological warfare scientists at Fort Detrick, Maryland. *Glasnost* brought a reversal of this propaganda tactic in late 1986 and an admission that the USSR also had cases of AIDS. Nelkin and Gilman emphasize that "blaming has always been a means to make mysterious and devastating diseases comprehensible and therefore possibly controllable" and that "perplexing medical questions have always generated hostility." Blaming becomes a political act, and many political leaders confuse medical goals with their ideological assumptions. Thus, exclusionary policies in the form of requiring testing for AIDS antibodies are directed at outsiders—in particular, at "immigrants, refugees, aliens, and even foreign students."

A variant of the cross-cultural implications of reactions to the AIDS pandemic is the ongoing controversy concerning the origins of the virus causing the disease. A particular source of resentment by Africans have been two theories, espoused by scientists writing in British scientific journals such as *The Lancet* and the *British Medical Journal*, summarized in American journals such as *Science* and *Scientific American*, and reiterated in press reports. The first theory is that AIDS has been endemic to Africa for a long time, perhaps for decades, but was unrecognized until the clustering of cases in recent years. The second is that HIV evolved from a virus found in African green monkeys and was somehow passed on to Africans and thence to the rest of the world. Both theories have been denounced as a residue of a colonialist mentality that sees Africa as both primitive and inferior. The African press generally rejected these theories and espoused the opposite view that AIDS had spread from Europe to Africa. Again, the article quoted above from *West Africa* excoriates the thesis that cases of AIDS in patients from Central Africa who are residing in Europe are proof that AIDS originated in Africa. Although many of these patients had been residing in Europe for a long time, the authors point out, the possibility that "they may have contracted the disease in Europe was not considered." The article concludes with this indictment:

> We would like to believe that the uncritical acceptance of the African connection was a simple error of judgement but it seems far more likely that the AIDS researchers, the medical experts, the media and the public at large are affected by the insidious and frequently unrecognized disease of racism (Chirimuuta et al. 1988:312).

One episode in this acrimonious debate is worth noting because of the light it sheds on cultural misperceptions and sensitivities. In an exchange of letters appearing in the *Scientific*

American, Muniini Mulera (1989), a Uganda-trained physician, denounced an article in the October 1988 issue, co-authored by Robert C. Gallo and Luc Montagnier. Gallo, of the National Cancer Institute in Bethesda, Maryland, and Montagnier, of the Pasteur Institute, Paris, had reiterated the premise that AIDS had been present in Central Africa for many years. Accusing the authors of ignorance of the demography and history of Central Africa, Mulera pointed out that the migration between city and countryside had been going on at least since the Second World War, that health services in Uganda were "excellent" from 1950 to the end of the 1970s, and that no cases of AIDS had been diagnosed before 1982. Citing a blood-sampling survey carried out between 1976 and 1984 which he believes repudiated the thesis that AIDS originated in Africa, he concluded that we do not know the origin of HIV, "but perpetuating a myth does not help science and only reinforces the ever-present racism and bigotry toward Africans" (10). Gallo and Montagnier replied that they had postulated that (1) the AIDS epidemic had begun in the United States, Haiti, and Central Africa at approximately the same time; (2) HIV has been present in humans for more than 100 years; (3) demographic changes may have spread the disease from smaller, closed groups to larger ones, creating new patterns of the disease; (4) cases were identified in retrospect in Central Africa as early as the 1960s; (5) high rates of infection were found among prostitutes in Rwanda in 1983; (6) retroviruses related to the human AIDS retroviruses were found in African monkeys but never in New World or Asian primates; and (7) the question of the origin of the AIDS virus is obviously related to but different from the factors that govern the epidemic in each region or area. The authors concluded:

> We do not suggest that the virus was transmitted en masse from central Africa to other areas or that the people of that region are any more responsible for the disease's transmission than, say, the residents of Connecticut are responsible for Lyme disease, which in fact was first described in Lyme, Conn. What we postulate as the trigger of the epidemic in central Africa—changing demography and behavior—is equally applicable to groups in Europe and the Americas. Historically we note that many microbes appear to have originated in Europe and the Americas or were first found in humans there.

We deeply regret, and in fact do not understand, an interpretation of our work and opinions on the origin of HIV that finds bigotry or suggests we blame anyone, much less an entire continent. In our opinion, HIV-1 very likely originated in a small region of central Africa and HIV-2 in western Africa. This point is not based on prejudice, nor is it purely academic; it has major long-term medical importance, and we believe it is time to discuss facts openly and honestly (Gallo & Montagnier 1989:11).

The positive response: The global mobilization against AIDS

Although the United Nations was slow to mobilize in the wake of the global threat of AIDS, in the first decade of the pandemic the UN system mounted what it described in its literature as one of the few genuinely international efforts in human history. Given the brief history of the pandemic, this development was characterized as extraordinary by Jonathan Mann (1988b). He identified three significant periods in the evolution of a global attack on AIDS.

The first, starting in the mid-1970s, was the time of the silent pandemic, during which the HIV infection spread—undetected, unrecognized—through five continents.

The second was a time of discovery, occurring, fortunately, at a time when scientific knowledge had developed the tools to detect human pathogens of the type that ultimately was identified as causing AIDS. The description of the AIDS syndrome in 1981 initiated another period of discovery during which the modes in which the disease was transmitted were defined, the specific causative virus was discovered, and the ability to identify antiviral antibodies was developed. In turn, the presence of antibodies to the HIV infection revealed that large numbers of individuals were infected—although asymptomatically—and that there was a long latency period between infection and the appearance of symptoms of the full-fledged disease. This new information was brought together and made public at the first international conference in 1985. Its effect, according to Mann, was to mark a dawning awareness of the broad impact of AIDS and to stir feelings of a powerful international solidarity.

The third period has been characterized by a global mobilization of scientific and public health resources against the pandemic through the establishment in February 1987 of a Special Programme on AIDS, under the leadership of WHO, later to be renamed the

Global Programme on AIDS (GPA).

The establishment of the program marked a turning point, as the Panos Dossier (1989:92–93) notes: "From this point on, the climate of world opinion on AIDS seemed to change almost overnight." Until then, national sensibilities prevailed; some countries would not acknowledge publicly that they were affected, for the reasons discussed above. Indeed, this continued to be the case throughout 1987, but "the tide had turned." The problem faced by WHO was to launch a massive effort on a global scale for which there had been few precedents. The campaign against smallpox, which was launched in 1967 and which is considered to have achieved its eradication in 1980, is such a precedent. The smallpox campaign cost $81 million. Obviously, the worldwide cost of the war on AIDS, impossible to calculate at this early stage, will be enormously greater.[3]

The World Health Organization Global Programme on AIDS

The principal role of the GPA is to coordinate national efforts at surveillance, prevention, and research, and to function as a resource for governments in their efforts to develop national control plans. Its three major avowed goals are (1) to halt the spread of the pandemic by preventing new HIV infections; (2) to provide support for individuals already infected; and (3) to unite national and international efforts to stem the tide of AIDS. The GPA coordinates worldwide surveillance; reports are received from WHO collaborating centers throughout the world as well as from individual ministries of health. By 1990, a total of 181 countries were reporting AIDS cases to what is, in effect, a global data bank.

The GPA developed into a fairly large organization, with sections devoted to program support, surveillance, health education, social and behavioral research, biomedical research, and epidemiological research (World Health Organization 1988). Coordinated by the GPA, both industrialized and developing countries have launched ambitious and aggressive prevention and control programs. The specific objectives of these efforts have been (1) to prevent sexual transmission of AIDS; (2) to screen blood and blood products; (3) to improve the sterilization of skin-piercing instruments; (4) to improve the management of HIV infection; and (5) to strengthen the monitoring and examination of data on AIDS. In implementing these

---

[3] For further details of the Global Programme on AIDS, see Chapter 8 of the Panos Dossier (1989).

activities, the GPA has facilitated, encouraged, or co-sponsored a number of regional conferences in Africa, the Americas, Southeast Asia, Europe, the eastern Mediterranean region, and the western Pacific, providing a mechanism for the exchange of expertise, field experience, and ideas for health professionals.

One signal accomplishment of the GPA, according to the Africanists Barnett and Blaikie (1992:17), has been the establishment of an AIDS database on both mortality and infection which—even if it is flawed—serves as a basis for developing national reporting systems and national AIDS policies.

One of the GPA's vital functions since its inception has been to alert the World Bank concerning the latest assessments of the future course of the pandemic. Under the leadership of Jonathan Mann, its first director, the organization became a catalyst for informing the world concerning the dangers of the pandemic and for launching programs to contain it. Mann championed a nontraditional public health approach to AIDS which transcended immediate concerns with the health aspects of the pandemic and which stressed the centrality of human rights in all its strategies. The distinguishing feature of the first phase of the GPA program has been a concern not only for the toll in human suffering and death but also for the social burden of stigma and the resulting discrimination against AIDS victims. The strategy of combating the disease itself went beyond distributing condoms to emphasizing a broader behavioral and social science approach, which included steering the GPA toward supporting nongovernmental organizations (NGOs) throughout the world.

In March 1990, Mann resigned from his position as director of the GPA, citing philosophical differences with his superior, Hiroshi Nakajima, the director general of WHO, who had cut the GPA budget—thus putting it on a more equal footing with other WHO programs. Under the leadership of Mann's successor, Michael Merson, also a public health physician, the GPA has changed in both style and direction. The style is more managerial, which some observers consider appropriate for consolidating and sustaining the GPA programs within the WHO bureaucracy. A more fundamental difference is a change in philosophy. Merson's objective is to warn those developing countries where the HIV virus has not yet established a bridgehead. He argues that if these vulnerable countries wait for AIDS cases to appear, "it is too darn late." He stresses a policy of encouraging condom use, developing targeted educational programs, and paying increased attention to the treatment of all sexually transmitted diseases. Under his administration, less attention is paid to the behavioral aspects of AIDS; funds for behavioral research have accordingly been reduced.

Mann takes issue with this narrower focus, arguing against the temptation to define away the pandemic by calling it a central problem of the industrialized world but just another endemic problem of the developing world. He argues against blaming those whose behavior is not changing rapidly enough, and he asserts that to wait "for technology to rescue us from ourselves" is tantamount to letting the pandemic dominate us (*Science,* News and Comment, October 25, 1991:512). The reality of the second phase of the GPA's stewardship is that in the second decade of the pandemic it faces the battle against AIDS with a reduced staff and reduced funds at a time when a concern with the international aspects no longer is front page news throughout the world.[4]

The annual AIDS conferences: An international forum

WHO provides the leadership for creating a unique international forum through annual conferences on AIDS which are co-sponsored by the WHO and host countries. It was through these conferences that the dimensions of the pandemic; its commonalties and diverse features; and its scientific, medical, social, economic, and cultural implications emerged. Each has attracted increasingly larger numbers of participants—epidemiologists, virologists, public health specialists, physicians, statisticians, and field workers in nongovernmental organizations—from around the world. Increasingly, the conferences have included social scientists, especially behavioral psychologists, demographers, economists, political scientists, and sociologists. And there is always a large international press corps in attendance.

The first international conference on AIDS was held in Atlanta, Georgia, in 1985. It was concerned primarily with scientific topics (molecular biology, virology, immunology, epidemiology, clinical medicine, and public health) and drew some 2,000 participants. It was at the second conference in Paris, in 1986, that news from the developing world revealed that AIDS was indeed an international problem without an immediate solution, requiring a global response.

---

[4] According to Earickson (1990), the growing pandemic coincides with a period of decreasing Western support for WHO and of decreasing U.S. support for its sister agency the Pan American Health Organization. The United States has thus far made only what has been called a modest contribution of funds to WHO earmarked for the AIDS program.

Realizing that progress toward developing vaccines for immunization as well as drugs for treatment would not take place in the
immediate future, the conference planners began to stress the social
aspects of AIDS.

The third conference in Washington in 1987 took on political
overtones. President Reagan, bowing to public pressure, delivered
a speech on AIDS the evening before the conference, and Vice
President Bush addressed the opening ceremony. Gay activist
groups began to draw attention to the human impact of the disease
through demonstrations outside the conference hall.

At the fourth conference, held in Stockholm in 1988 and
attended by over 7,000 people, the program not only stressed
humanitarian concerns for the victims of the disease but also
identified emerging social, ethical, and legal implications.

At the fifth conference, held in Montreal in 1989 and attended
by 11,000 people, conflict between activist groups—agitating for
more rapid U.S government action in research and treatment and
the conference organizers became quite apparent. The sessions of
the conference named "AIDS, Society, and Behaviour" reflected
these social concerns. Individual panels discussed the impact of
AIDS on the individual and on families, the ethics of testing for HIV,
the role of religion and the media, the problems of AIDS in the
workplace, the impact of AIDS on minorities, and patients' rights to
privacy—among a host of topics demonstrating the social implications of the pandemic.

The need to respond to the changing nature of the concern for
AIDS was echoed by Alastair Clayton (1989), director general of the
Canadian Federal Centre for AIDS, as the Montreal conference
began. Noting that some 70 percent of the abstracts submitted were
biomedical, he said he would like the ratio to be 50–50. The signal
distinguishing characteristic of each successive conference, however, has been the inclusion and increasing recognition of the roles
of PWAs (persons with AIDS) and organized gay activist groups.
Robert Wachtler (1991), a physician AIDS specialist who was one of
the principal organizers of the 1990 San Francisco conference,
refers to the preceding Montreal conference as a landmark of the
activist movement. It was at Montreal, he observes, that the activists
"exploded." In planning the next conference in San Francisco, he
reports, the increasingly formidable presence of these activist
groups in the newly created field of AIDS politics was a dominant
concern.

The 1990 San Francisco conference may have represented the
peak of the emphasis on community and policy issues, but the focal

issue that emerged during the months of planning that preceded it was an international one. Wachtler describes how the barring of a Dutch delegate to the conference under the U.S. immigration rule prohibiting seropositives from entering the country became a rally-ing point for opposition to the law.

Opposition to the ban on seropositives became the focus of international criticism of the U.S. policy. On November 23, 1989, the International Red Cross announced its intention to boycott the San Francisco conference. Despite a subsequent waiver in visa proce-dures that permitted seropositive travelers to attend the conference if they admitted being infected and accepted having their passport stamped with this information, the boycott was joined by the International AIDS Society, the World Hemophilia Association, the governments of France and Switzerland, and ultimately the Euro-pean Community. As Wachtler reports, the discriminatory travel policy offered Europeans, and especially the French, the opportu-nity to "wrap themselves in the flag of righteousness and elevate the travel restriction issue to a test of moral integrity" (145). The U.S. national organization of PWAs also joined the boycott.[5] In response, the Department of Health and Human Services and the Immigration and Naturalization Service amended the wording of the travel restriction to avoid documentation of the applicant's status and thus to protect the confidentiality of this information.

Yielding to further international and domestic pressures, the Department of Justice[6] issued a travel plan exempting individuals who applied for a ten-day stay to attend the conference from revealing their HIV status—"in the public interest." This compro-mise effectively lifted the boycott of attendance at the San Francisco conference.

The seventh AIDS conference was held in Florence, Italy, in 1991. Observers at the conference, which had 8,000 participants, noted a sea change in the tone of the event. The conference was primarily scientific in nature, showing a reduced emphasis on sessions devoted to social policy issues and an increased sense of failure at efforts in education and behavior change (*New York Times*,

---

[5] On December 12, 1989, June Osborn, as chair of the U.S. National Commission on AIDS, labeled the restrictions "counterproductive, discrimi-natory, and a waste of resources . . . They reinforce the false impression that AIDS and HIV infection are a general threat when in fact they are sharply restricted in their mode of transmission" (quoted in Wachtler 1991:119).

[6] The Immigration and Naturalization Service is a component of the Depart-ment of Justice.

June 17, 1991:7). The Bush administration's decision to finance the travel of only half the number of scientists originally scheduled to attend was criticized by attending scientists from all over the world.[7] The Italian chairman of the conference stressed that the exchange of ideas among scientists was a crucial aspect of the meeting and he noted that the participants would sorely miss the opportunities for discussions with the absent American scientists.

Some participants at the Florence conference launched sharp attacks on the U.S. government's continuing policy of restricting the entry of infected travelers. Organizers of the next conference, which was scheduled to be sponsored by Harvard University and convened in Boston in 1992, warned that they would cancel the conference, in response to the mounting criticism, if the restrictions were not removed.[8] The European Community again expressed its concern over the restrictions. But an undercurrent of questioning by an increasing number of scientists concerning the costs and value of the conferences was also evident. In fact, in recent years more scientists have chosen to release their research findings to professional journals rather than in presentations at these conferences. However, Anthony Fauci of the U.S. National Institute of Allergy and Infectious Disease, the ranking U.S. government scientist at the Florence conference, voiced disappointment that more U.S scientists had not been able to attend and noted that some scientists had funded their own travel (*New York Times*, June 17, 1991:7).

At the conference, Jonathan Mann voiced the criticism that the international AIDS program was being affected by complacency and foot dragging and he called for a renewal of the international response. He also criticized the lack of papers on the social impact of AIDS. According to Oliver Morton, the science editor of *The Economist*, "in Florence, the sense of urgency that was common to all the previous conferences seems to have faded. It is not gone . . . But it is not the progressive force it once was" (quoted in *AIDS & Society*, July/August 1991:2).

---

[7] The U.S. government supported the attendance of more than 700 scientists at the San Francisco conference. It reduced that number to 400 for the Florence meeting because of travel costs. New budget restrictions imposed by the Congress subsequently forced the Public Health Service to cut the 400 figure in half.

[8] Commenting on the continuing AIDS ban, an editorial in the *New York Times* (June 19, 1991:A24) stated that it is a "travesty that the United States, with one of the largest AIDS-infected populations in the world, has taken a stance that implies the danger comes from abroad."

In August 1991, the Harvard AIDS Institute, the organizers of the planned 1992 Boston conference, announced that because of the travel restrictions it was canceling the conference. In September, it was announced that the conference would be held in Amsterdam; the Netherlands had no HIV-related restrictions on travel or immigration (*Science*, Briefings, September 27, 1991:1484). In the official announcement, the Harvard-Amsterdam organizers stated that the goal of the conference would be to present new results of basic, clinical, and epidemiological research and to help strengthen understanding of the social dimensions of the epidemic.

The Amsterdam AIDS conference, held July 19–22, 1992, was the largest thus far; it was attended by some 12,000 individuals.[9] It was also expensive, costing $25 million according to some reports. The day before it opened, an editorial in *The Lancet*, deploring this expense, declared that "the era of mega-conferences [on AIDS] should now end" ("AIDS: An Opportunity Not to Be Lost" 1992:148).

The highlights of the Amsterdam conference were public policy issues: human rights, women and AIDS, the role of nongovernmental organizations (NGOs) in the developing world's struggle against AIDS, and the emerging roles of organizations of persons with AIDS (PWAs)—issues that had largely been left hanging in Montreal. For the first time, women's issues received focused attention. The inclusion of activists in the program made protests less disruptive than in the past: most of the protests were aimed at the shortcomings of the U.S. government's leadership in HIV-AIDS issues. The discovery of a possible "new virus" dominated the scientific sessions and captured the attention of the international press.

Press reports of the conference referred to a pervading feeling of pessimism concerning the future—a pessimism that had first become manifest at the Florence conference. As Lawrence K. Altman, the physician-reporter of the *New York Times* noted, the conference ended on a somber note, generated by the growing recognition that "AIDS is yielding its secrets slowly and . . . the full dimensions of the puzzle are not known" (*New York Times*, July 26, 1992:1).

Critics of the Amsterdam conference stressed the fact that 85 percent of the participants came from the industrialized countries.

---

[9] The eighth international conference on AIDS was held in conjunction with the STD World Congress and was sponsored by Harvard University and the Dutch AIDS Foundation; co-sponsors were the International AIDS Society and WHO.

In the words of one observer, the conference was "the regional meeting of the North" (Berkley 1992:3).

A more trenchant and radical criticism was voiced by the Australian Dennis Altman (1993:7), who, following the Amsterdam conference, complained that the international AIDS conferences "are largely U.S. national conferences, at which the rest of us are often onlookers." American predominance is not confined to scientists and doctors but includes activists as well. "Western and non-western community activists do not for the most part share the same priorities," he added. Furthermore, he noted, "the issues around AIDS in the rich world are increasingly driven by the latest developments in medical technology, which is irrelevant to the great majority of those infected in the developing world." In order for the developing world to be heard at these conferences, Altman believes, national quotas will have to be imposed to prevent the domination of any one country's agenda.

The ninth international conference on AIDS was held in Berlin, June 7–11, 1993, and drew 14,000 participants. This conference also sounded an alarm concerning the unchecked spread of the AIDS virus throughout the world. Again, the dominant note was pessimism concerning the rate of scientific progress in dealing with HIV infection and AIDS disease. Lawrence Altman, in summarizing the conference for the *New York Times* (June 12, 1993:5), quoted Michael Merson as saying that "we must accept that our scientific advances today are coming in small steps, not in leaps and bounds."

Scientists working on the development of a vaccine reported new obstacles. The AIDS virus is ever-changing: five, perhaps six major genetic subtypes of the main virus (HIV-1) have been identified. Moreover, different subtypes of HIV predominate in different parts of the world, only to be replaced by other, mutating strains that become dominant. This phenomenon has already been observed in Thailand and in South America. The Swedish epidemiologist Lars O. Kallings raised the possibility that in developing a vaccine, scientists may need to monitor HIV as they now do the influenza virus, adjusting the vaccine periodically to target the latest mutations.

News presented at the meeting about the effectiveness of anti-HIV drugs was also disheartening. A large-scale European study whose results questioned the value of using AZT to delay the onset of AIDS symptoms in HIV-infected people had been made public a month before the conference and had been criticized by American physicians. At the conference, additional data on the design of the study satisfied many critics.

Summarizing the conference, Altman wrote that only "an eternal optimist" would have left the meetings believing that new drugs would be available in time to save the lives of the 14 million people now infected throughout the world or that a vaccine would be developed in time to prevent the infection of the more than 30 million people predicted by the year 2000 (*New York Times*, June 15, 1993:C-1). The one clear note sounded at Berlin is that the only hope of stemming the pandemic at this time is through prevention.

The international AIDS conferences have come under attack from critics who claim they are counterproductive because of their huge size and circus-like atmosphere. On the eve of the Berlin conference, the British journal *Nature* called for their end, as *The Lancet* had done a year earlier before the Amsterdam conference. Kallings, however, speaking in Berlin, defended the conferences, maintaining that they serve a vital function because of the degree of involvement of both persons with AIDS (PWAs) and scientists—a feature that distinguishes them from other conferences that exclude patients from their conceptualization and planning. The question, Kallings said, is whether the next meeting in Yokohama in 1994 will report examples of how policies for preventing the spread of the epidemic have been changed and proof that these efforts have reduced high-risk behavior.

Critique of the global response

The continuing escalation of the AIDS pandemic has ushered in a critical evaluation of international efforts to control it. The critique came to a head in 1992 with the publication of a book edited by Jonathan Mann, Daniel J. M. Tarantola, and Thomas W. Neller, *AIDS in the World*, which surveys AIDS programs throughout the world.[10] Their results contradict a number of optimistic accounts of the global response. The gist of the Harvard group's critique follows.

The world mobilization against AIDS, which started in 1986–87, drew on scientific progress to create a rapidly growing knowledge of the epidemiology of HIV/AIDS and its behavioral and cultural origins. But in the 1990s the disease continues to spread rapidly, while the attack against it does not keep pace (Mann et al. 1992:841). The course of the pandemic throughout the world is not being affected in any serious manner at either the national or the

---

10 The editors are members of the Global AIDS Policy Coalition of the International AIDS Center, Harvard AIDS Institute, Harvard School of Public Health.

international level. So far, the Harvard critics maintain, there has been a failure to mobilize and respond as a unified global community to a common threat. At the beginning of the second decade of AIDS this failure raises this question: "Is the global epidemic out of control?" Here are some specific criticisms:[11]

- The global response to the threat of HIV infection and AIDS disease is inadequate and uncoordinated at both national and international levels. It is a threatening "collective failure."
- In thirteen of the thirty-seven countries surveyed, the head of state has still not spoken publicly about AIDS. In another thirteen countries, the first statement by the head of state was not made until 1989 or later.
- Inadequacies in program response can be found in both industrialized and developing countries where counseling is not offered systematically and where socially disadvantaged persons lack access to prevention advice and care facilities.
- Experience at the community level during a decade of experience shows that HIV prevention is entirely possible, but only where information and education programs and health and social services are available and where there is a supportive social environment. Programs aimed at homosexual men, intravenous drug users, prostitutes, and adolescents have all increased knowledge and produced behavioral change. But these pilot programs are hampered by a lack of resources and the failure to extend them to larger groups.
- National AIDS programs are too narrowly conceived as governmental or official programs. To succeed, they must combine the efforts of government, nongovernmental organizations. and the private sector.
- One third of all national AIDS programs have never been evaluated, and program managers have been

---

[11] This summary is abstracted from Chapter 1 of *AIDS in the World*, "A Global Epidemic out of Control?" A similar assessment was voiced earlier by David E. Rogers, vice chair of the U.S. National Commission on AIDS, who stated in an editorial in the *American Journal of Public Health* : "We are deep into a disaster of unprecedented worldwide proportions and too many people are sitting passively on the sidelines watching it unfold" (Rogers 1992:522).

replaced after two years in two-thirds of the programs studied.
- Global spending by industrialized countries for HIV prevention and AIDS care in the developing world has declined from $140 million a year since 1991. Only 6 percent of total spending for HIV prevention was in the developing world. Wealthy nations are showing a growing preference to work independently, on a bilateral basis, with developing countries at the same time that international organizations are finding it difficult to agree on allocating responsibility and coordinating their efforts. The HIV/AIDS menace is increasingly perceived as a developing country problem.

In effect, the Harvard group maintains that, after a decade of mobilization, the response in the second decade of the pandemic has reached a plateau.[12] In impassioned terms, the editors speak of the need for "a new vision," a global perspective:

A global vision of AIDS is as important to the local, national, and international future as is global thinking about the Earth's physical environment. Indeed, if we were unaware how interdependent our world has become in the past twenty-five years—in political, economic, and social terms—AIDS would have taught us this great lesson (Mann et al. 1992:2).

A rationale for international collaboration

Nicholas A. Christakis (1990:329), a public health physician, identifies the common interests and divergent needs that mandate an international response. "Unlike other so-called international health problems, such as malaria and smallpox," he points out, "AIDS strikes the developing and developed world with equal vengeance and forces all nations to consider their common interests in the solution of international health problems." The AIDS pandemic, he notes, "provides a new opportunity to view health as an international phenomenon, one that is best addressed by policies with international dimensions" (329).

---

[12] For example, the 1992 AIDS budget for WHO was $90 million, in contrast to $110 million the previous year.

In identifying AIDS as an international health problem, Christakis raises the following questions: Which aspects of the spread of the disease need international attention? What should the national and international objectives of AIDS control be? Why should the international impact of AIDS concern single nations? Why, for example, should the United States be interested in devoting efforts to control AIDS elsewhere rather than in concentrating solely on its own epidemic? One answer to these questions is that AIDS is a pandemic, and a pandemic disease cannot be addressed in the same manner as an epidemic disease. AIDS transcends national boundaries in the sense that it occurs worldwide. Yet the fact of worldwide occurrence in itself does not make it an international problem:

> There is a distinction between a *worldwide* problem and an *international* problem. The latter has an important feature in addition to worldwide occurrence. This feature is the direct interrelatedness of the problem in one country with the problem in another or of the cause of the problem in one country with the effect in another (Christakis 1990:330).

In this sense AIDS is typical of other international problems such as pollution, ozone depletion, arms proliferation, and hunger. All of these require international approaches. By the same token, "narrow, nationalistic" policies directed at controlling the spread of AIDS are not effective.

A host of factors arising out of the increasing interdependence of the modern world are contributing to the spread of AIDS and make an international approach to control essential. Among these are the immigration and travel of HIV-infected individuals, trade in defective condoms and antibody testing kits, international transport of HIV-infected blood, and the interdiction of illegal intravenous drugs (334). None of these factors can be controlled unilaterally: international cooperative efforts are essential to improve the basic health care infrastructure of developing countries. In this context, Christakis notes that even if an effective vaccine against AIDS were eventually to be developed, inadequate public health infrastructures in developing countries would militate against its effective worldwide utilization.

International collaboration is also crucial to advancing scientific research on AIDS. Researchers see sub-Saharan Africa as an ideal site for human research trials of AIDS vaccines and drugs for both practical and scientific reasons, especially the low labor costs and the availability of large study populations. Trials of a vaccine, for example, would require research subjects who are free of HIV infection but at risk of such infection, a requirement easier to meet in Africa than in the developed world. Trials of drugs for treating AIDS require "pharmacologically virgin" subjects, that is, individuals who do not self-medicate with putative anti-HIV agents. Such subjects are more common in Africa than in the United States and Europe. Zalduondo et al. (1990) make a similar point when they note that it is questionable whether the appropriate testing of an AIDS vaccine—should one be developed—could be successfully carried out without international cooperation.

Christakis warns that, although some of the stakes raised by the AIDS pandemic are international in character and require international cooperative effort, other aspects of the AIDS problem can only be managed effectively by national efforts. Indeed, when international organizations coordinate some national efforts or are involved in delivering local care, they often overlook local sociocultural issues. For this reason, the WHO global program on AIDS fosters national initiatives to control AIDS that are in keeping with international goals.

Common interests in fighting AIDS bind the nations of the world in a close confederation of international effort, but a host of divergent interests mandate different approaches. Perhaps the most disparate are in the major loci of infection in the world—the United States, one of the most developed regions in the world, and Central Africa, one of the least developed.

These are social rather than medical problems, and for these, Christakis maintains, an international approach is less useful. One such problem is sexuality, which is deeply embedded in local cultural traditions. Prostitution, a major contributor to AIDS, Christakis holds, is likely to have a different dynamic in Paris, Rio de Janeiro, Port au Prince, New York, and Kinshasa, and thus requires different control strategies. Moreover, national research agendas—particularly in the field of social science research on the spread of HIV infection, on intravenous drug use, and on sexual behavior in different parts of the world—are bound to differ. But while the specific aspects of the problem of combating AIDS may differ, all nations, according to Christakis, are motivated by an interest in controlling the disease—beyond its threat to health—because of its potential threat to the very structure of society.

A growing number of analysts have concluded that the social

consequences of AIDS, as much as the causes of AIDS, have both common origins and divergent manifestations and require international collaboration in sharing experience, insights, and approaches to solutions.

A number of aspects of the AIDS pandemic are crucial to its understanding. First is the special trauma resulting from AIDS attacks against specific subgroups in societies throughout the world—young adults, the disadvantaged, ethnic minorities, and the children who are victims of congenital AIDS and whose drug-addicted mothers are equally doomed. Second is the strain imposed on health services that deal with these groups—in rich countries like the United States as well as in the economically deprived developing countries. Third are the ubiquitous expressions of prejudice and the practice of discrimination in the workplace against individuals suspected of being carriers. Fourth, we must consider a host of issues that have surfaced since AIDS began to exact its human toll: for example, devising control measures in penal situations, in the military, in public schools. Finally, certain ethical issues are becoming manifest as a result of the clash between individual rights to privacy and the interest of society in protecting itself against the spread of the disease.

Speaking from the standpoint of a sociologist, Richard Rockwell (1988:5223) articulated a further rationale for examining the social implications of AIDS. "Even if no one else is ever again infected," he maintained, "the pandemic will have historically significant consequences. The lethal virus does not have to kill in hundreds of millions before we see social impacts beyond the lives it takes, and the social and economic burden their illnesses and deaths impose."

5

Public Reactions

The Relevance of History

As the full extent of the AIDS phenomenon became evident during the 1980s, the press and the other media—especially in the United States—were filled with speculations about the future and with comparisons with other epidemics in the past. In 1987, for example, an interview with former Secretary of Health and Human Services Otis R. Bowen was headlined as "AIDS May Dwarf the Plague" in the *New York Times* (January 30, 1987:A24).[1] This particular incident fueled press and media interest in superficial historical comparisons; the concept of AIDS as a "plague" was reinforced.[2] Historians Elizabeth Fee and Daniel M. Fox (1988) remark that many colleagues had been asked by reporters to encapsulate in a sentence or two the history of social response to epidemics. And Rosenkrantz (1988), a historian of science, noted that she is frequently asked if there are historical precedents for the

---

[1] An even more pessimistic comparison was made by Halfdan Mahler, former director-general of the World Health Organization, who, when asked to compare AIDS to other epidemics, such as smallpox, said he could not think of anything else that matched the estimates that 100 million people would be infected with AIDS within ten years of its discovery (quoted in McLaughlin 1989:15).

[2] The term plague is used loosely in common parlance and particularly in the context of AIDS. As William H. Foege (1988), a public health physician, noted, even the medical definition of plague is fraught with ambiguity. The 1986 *Webster's Medical Desk Dictionary* describes plague as an epidemic disease causing a high rate of mortality, a definition that has been superseded.

AIDS epidemic.

Antedating the journalistic interest in metaphors that would provide graphic comparisons for a frightening and mysterious disease are articles in scholarly journals that sought to examine AIDS in historical perspective. Historians of medicine and public health, research scientists, and sociologists have all looked for parallels and distinguishing contrasts between AIDS and other pandemics of the past. Indeed, as Fee and Fox (1988:1) note, AIDS "has stimulated more interest in history than any other disease of modern times."

The relevance of history is that detailed historical analysis of the meaning and impact of fulminating mass disease throughout history—as distinct from the search for facile metaphors and analogies—can provide an invaluable perspective on the current AIDS crisis. As Allan M. Brandt, a historian of medicine, underscores, an understanding of the past may help inform our assessment of contemporary health problems. In his preface to a book on the social history of venereal disease (1987:vii), he states that "only when we recognize that diseases have a social history—that they are more than discrete biological entities and that their causes are complex and varied, will we be able to address them effectively and humanely."

The value of examining the history of disease for understanding the present-day AIDS phenomenon is based on four fundamental premises:

1. There are universal and timeless aspects in group human reactions to lethal disease on a massive scale.

2. These reactions are determined in large measure by how disease has been perceived or defined and how this perception is culturally determined.

3. Societies' responses to the threatened outbreak of epidemic disease, that is, the organized, official

---

Epidemiologists now use the term epidemic to describe "an unusual occurrence of a disease or condition." Thus, while a single case of smallpox might be labeled an "epidemic," the million cases of gonorrhea each year in the United States would be considered an endemic disease and not necessarily an epidemic. Foege points to two problems with the Webster's definition: (1) plagues do not have to be epidemic: a "plague can be endemic, a constant presence," and (2) "mortality rates should not be the criterion for measurement" (333). The definition of the word has "enlarged," and he suggests that a better working definition would be "a disease or other condition causing high mortality or morbidity and often accompanied by social dislocation" (334).

efforts of communities to control the spread of infection, are influenced both by how the disease has been perceived and by public fear of contagion.

4.   Mass epidemics have pervasive social consequences that transcend the immediate, visible toll of suffering and death.

Rosenberg (1990), a sociologist, addresses the first premise by stating that understanding our current reactions to AIDS depends on distinguishing the universal aspects of behavior—as revealed by public reactions to past episodic outbreaks of deadly disease—from the aspects that are unique to our time. Medical historian Risse (1988) advances a cogent reason for this analysis: we are already repeating these reactions, he says, despite our sophistication.

Addressing the second premise, Brandt (1988a) states that the principal task in examining the historical record for relevant contemporary insights is to learn how people have perceived, or defined, the scourges of the past. His thesis, and that of other historians and social scientists (Fox 1988a; Keniston 1990; Rosenberg 1988a), biologists (Lederberg 1988), and physicians (Thomas 1988), is that a disease is not only a biological phenomenon but a social one as well. Dominant beliefs, cultural values, and social expectations shape the manner in which diseases are viewed over time. In this sense, diseases can be said to be "socially constructed."

The third premise, that is, that the social construction of epidemic disease influences, affects, and shapes official response measures designed to control the spread of infection, leads historians to stress the value of the lessons of history. As Brandt (1988b) points out, "throughout human history, epidemic disease has constituted a natural experiment in how societies respond to disability, dependence, fear, and death." This, in turn, reveals society's "most fundamental cultural, social, and moral values" (414–415). More immediately, significant implications for public policy on AIDS can be gleaned from history (McKinlay et al. 1989).

The fourth premise, which deals with the social impact of epidemics, has been a recent concern of social historians. The social history of the major catastrophic outbreaks of disease that have occurred throughout the world from medieval times to the present has documented the influence of disease not only on the course of contemporary events but also on the very structure of society. William H. McNeill's classic, *Plagues and People* (1976), contains extensive documentation of this influence, particularly for the premodern period. Swenson (1988), a physician and microbiologist, outlines how plagues have affected aspects of history as diverse as the balance of power, changes in class structure, religious leadership, and the economy. Other observers have focused on the impact of epidemic diseases on the military (Brandt 1988c), on public health authority (Musto 1988; Slack 1988), and on science and medicine (Lederberg 1988; Thomas 1988). In short, the history of the social impact of epidemic disease—on the institutions that are the framework of society and on the actions involved in combating virulent outbreaks, which are as important as the epidemiological record of morbidity and mortality—provides a singularly relevant context for understanding the complexities of the unfolding AIDS story.

The list of catastrophic diseases that have invited comparison with AIDS is a long one; included here are both pandemics and localized but nonetheless devastating epidemics.

Major pandemics

The bubonic plague, a bacterial infection transmitted by fleas from rats to humans, has become an immortal metaphor for widespread and deadly disease. The plague had numerous outbreaks in ancient Greece, in the Middle East, and in Europe in the premodern era. What may have been the first pandemic, known as the Justinian plague, caused the death of 20 to 25 percent of the population of the Roman Empire. Major outbreaks occurred in the seventh century. Between 1347 and 1351, what became graphically described as the "Black Death" swept across Europe. Striking indiscriminately at all ages and classes, it caused the death of one-third of the population.

Repeated occurrences of plague continued to cause mortality on a similar scale throughout the next three centuries, although the disease was largely concentrated in towns and cities. Padua lost half its population in 1405 and Milan half in 1680; Genoa lost 60 percent in ten years; Norwich, England in 1579, Venice in 1630, Marseilles in 1720, and Moscow in 1771 each successively lost about 30 percent of its citizens (Simpson 1988; Slack 1988; Swensen 1988).

The cholera pandemic of the nineteenth century rivaled the bubonic plague in its diffusion. Indeed, its outreach was even greater, for it covered three continents. Originating in India in 1817, it swept into Russia in 1830 and reached Mecca and Europe a year later. Subsequently, it crossed the Atlantic.

The United States experienced three cholera epidemics in the nineteenth century. Breaking out first in Canada in the spring of 1832, cholera swept south, reached New Orleans, which had 5,000 cases, and westward to Oregon. In New York City, the epidemic killed 3,500 people before it ended. Subsequent smaller epidemics occurred in 1849 and 1866. About half of the victims of cholera died (Risse 1988).

The most recent pandemic, until the advent of AIDS, was that of influenza in the early twentieth century. Caused by a virus, the victims succumbed to a secondary infection of pneumonia. First recognized in 1918 at an army post in Kansas, it soon broke out in Europe, striking Spain, France, and England. The infection was rapidly lethal: 700 people died in London alone in a three-week period, 53,000 cases occurred in Switzerland in the month of July. Some 5,100 people died within a two-week period in October in Philadelphia. It erupted in both India and Africa. By the time it ended, there had been about 550,000 deaths in the United States, 20 million in India, and an estimated 30 to 40 million throughout the world. The number of Americans who died surpassed the combined U.S. battle deaths in World War I, World War II, Korea, and Vietnam (Crosby 1989:207).

Major epidemics

The history of mass occurrences of disease includes major epidemics that have been geographically less extensive than the pandemics but that have been no less virulent and socially disruptive. Like the pandemics, they provide insights into their role as major actors in historical events, into how society has perceived their implied threats, how it has reacted to the crises, and how it took action to combat the plagues.

In the sixteenth century, a devastating epidemic of smallpox, a disease caused by a virus, was introduced into the New World by the Spanish conquistadors. The disease had been established in Europe before 1500, and the population had gradually developed immunity to it. Spaniards based in Cuba, themselves immune, introduced the disease to vulnerable native populations in Mexico in 1520. From there it spread to Central and South America, breaking out frequently in the sixteenth century. Killing from 15 to 18 million of a population of 25 million, as Swenson (1988) notes, the disease was a major factor in the ability of the Spanish to conquer the Americas.

Typhus played a major role in history early in the eighteenth century. Localized in Poland and Russia, it greeted Napoleon's armies in the 1812 invasion. By 1813, only 3,000 men of the 500,000 soldiers in the invading army were alive and completed the retreat. "The vast majority of deaths," notes Swenson," were the result of typhus and dysentery rather than battle injuries or exposure to the severe Russian winter" (1988:187).

Historians of medicine sometimes refer to the prevalence of tuberculosis in Europe from 1700 to 1870 as an "epidemic," although the characteristics of the disease differed from other epidemic diseases. It was a long-term illness that, before the advent of antibiotics in modern times, was almost invariably fatal. Its victims remained ambulatory for years, while being potentially infectious. In 1900, TB was the most frequent cause of death in the Western world, equaling today's death rates from cancer and accidents combined (Musto 1988).

Yellow fever, an acute, epidemic disease caused by a virus transmitted by the bite of a mosquito, caused repeated onslaughts in most cities in the United States and the Caribbean. When Philadelphia was the U.S. capital in 1793, it was struck by a yellow fever epidemic that caused governmental authorities to flee. It struck Natchez in 1823 and New Orleans in 1853, where it killed 10 percent of the population. It became one of the main obstacles to be overcome in the construction of the Panama Canal in the years prior to its formal opening in 1915.

Poliomyelitis (infantile paralysis), an acute viral infection, was both endemic and epidemic in all parts of the world, but it rarely occurred in the United States until 1907, after which time there were periodic outbreaks. From 1910 to 1914, there were 30,000 cases, with 5,000 deaths. New York City was struck in 1916, and periodic incursions occurred until the widespread use of the Salk vaccine in the 1950s (Risse 1988).

Syphilis, caused by a spirochete, is one of the most virulent of venereal diseases; it first surfaced in Spain in the fifteenth century. Reputedly introduced by sailors returning from the New World, it spread to France and Italy. Transmitted through sexual contact, it is a "smoldering illness" passed on by mothers to their fetuses during pregnancy. By the beginning of World War I, it was perceived as an epidemic. The apparent conquest of syphilis finally came about through the discovery of penicillin. During the 1950s, however, there was a recrudescence of the disease; despite the availability of the modern "magic bullet" of antibiotics, syphilis still has by no means been eliminated (Brandt 1987).

AIDS: An epidemiological comparison

Since AIDS invites comparison with other pandemics and epidemics, it is important to examine which of its characteristics biologists, clinicians, public health physicians, and social scientists have selected as unique or as similar to other catastrophic diseases. The answer to the question of how AIDS compares with other epidemic diseases has many components.

Viewed primarily as a biomedical phenomenon, AIDS is like no other epidemic disease because of its complicated pathology—a combination of successive immune dysfunctions that reveal themselves through the symptoms of a range of opportunistic infections that may vary in different settings. Joshua Lederberg (1988) focuses on another key distinguishing feature, namely, that those who are infected with HIV develop antibodies without acquiring immunity. In fact, they may go on to develop progressively more symptoms until the immune system collapses. The long incubation period, however, greatly increases opportunities to spread the infection to others. Keniston (1990) also stresses as a distinctive feature of AIDS the initial invisibility of the disease to its victims during the symptom-free interval after initial infection.

Hamburg and Fauci (1990:44), research scientists at the National Institutes of Health, stress the complicated etiology of AIDS that makes it a unique research problem. "The more knowledge is accumulated about the virus and the disease it produces," they observe, "the more complex the picture becomes." Indeed, AIDS researchers have subsequently been confronted with the fact that they are dealing with a mutating virus that confounds their efforts. Aron Ron and David E. Rogers (1990:108), both physicians, note how AIDS differs significantly from earlier epidemics, when neither the cause nor the methods of prevention were known. Instead, AIDS was swiftly recognized because it appeared at a time of "remarkable advances in biological research and increasing sophistication of disease surveillance systems." With AIDS, the cause and the means of transmission are known.[3] As an editorial in *Science* notes (Jasny 1993), the rate of progress in identifying HIV and understanding its life cycle and molecular biology are unprecedented. Ironically, however, according to a survey of 150 leading AIDS researchers conducted by *Science*, this knowledge is undermining assumptions

---

[3] Implementing control methods is the crucial problem. Controlling the spread of the epidemic is at present limited to education and behavioral change (Craven 1989).

held with confidence just a year earlier. In AIDS research, more knowledge leads to less certainty (*Science*, AIDS Research, May 28, 1993). And as Lawrence Altman, reporting from the 1993 Berlin AIDS conference pointed out, for HIV-infected patients this wealth of scientific knowledge contrasts sharply with the poverty of the clinical benefits it has yielded (*New York Times*, June 6, 1993:20).

The virologist William H. Haseltine (1990) has underscored the fact that HIV infection is lifelong and requires the continuing administration of antiviral drugs. In his speech to the French Academy of Sciences (Haseltine 1992:IV19), he succinctly described the mutability of the virus: "It changes as it grows." It is for this reason that it has been difficult to achieve long-lasting immune protection. "We do not know in which field of research a breakthrough may come," he said.

AIDS is unlike any other epidemic disease in the selectivity of its targets: that is, young people and persons in their prime productive and reproductive years (Armstrong & Bos 1992). As Gerald H. Friedland, a clinician who is co-director of the AIDS Center at the Montefiore Medical Center in New York, writes, "although familiar in developing countries, death on this scale in this age group, except during a war, is something we are not accustomed to . . . Death belongs to the old, not the young. AIDS causes an inversion of the expected life cycle . . . In areas like New York City, the numbers alone are both numbing and overwhelming . . . It is dozens and dozens of young men and women, in an increasing torrent over a very short period of time" (1990:133).

The physician David E. Rogers has pointed out another difference between AIDS and earlier plagues. Despite the horror and magnitude of the medieval bubonic plagues, of the influenza pandemic of 1918–19, and of the summer outbreaks of poliomyelitis in the developed countries that continued into the 1950s, these plagues at least were self-limiting. After a few years, for a variety of reasons, the rate of new infections would subside. Instead, AIDS is a truly persistent global pandemic; "it will be the plague of our professional lifetimes," Rogers writes, "and probably that of our children's lives as well" (1992:523).

For Jonathan Mann and his colleagues at Harvard (1992:4), the uniqueness of AIDS is that it is "a disease of human groups—

families, households, couples—and its demographic and social impacts multiply from the infected individual to the group." Furthermore, "no insects, food, or water mediate between the virus and humanity. Everywhere in the world, HIV spreads through the same basic and narrowly circumscribed routes of transmission—sex, blood, and mother-to-fetus/infant" (18).

AIDS is unique among epidemics in another aspect of selectivity: it strikes largely at subgroups in the population that are explicitly "at risk." So far, as noted earlier, it is present in selective clusters of infection in large urban centers. But most Americans, Rosenberg (1990:12) points out, have so far been largely spectators of the epidemic, which is a "media reality, both exaggerated and diminished as it is articulated in forms suitable for mass consumption." In contrast, the bubonic plague, for example, struck relatively uniformly throughout the entire population—as did cholera. The lasting effect of the AIDS pandemic, Rosenberg says, will not be in terms of sheer numbers of lives lost but rather in the nature of its social manifestations and their consequences—an assessment shared by most social historians searching the past for relevant parallels.

On the other hand, AIDS shares certain features with other epidemics. Like polio and influenza, the initial infection is followed by devastating symptoms (Keniston 1990). For the physician Lewis Thomas, AIDS is, "in plain fact, . . . a singularly contagious venereal disease" (1989:115). As a sexually transmitted disease, AIDS is most akin to venereal syphilis (Brandt 1988d) and hepatitis B.[4] For Keniston, a psychologist, this very similarity is cause for pessimism and dims the hope of eliminating AIDS. Despite the current availability of relatively inexpensive and nontoxic cures for syphilis, the ease with which it can be recognized and treated, and the existence of public health measures to trace and contact infected sexual partners, Keniston states, syphilis infection is still with us and will probably exist as a health threat for all foreseeable futures.[5] As an

---

[4] Hepatitis B is a nonlethal endemic infection which shares some characteristics with AIDS. Like AIDS, it is spread through infected blood, blood products, and sexual contact. As with AIDS, the agent of infection is a virus. There are about 200 million carriers throughout the world, mostly in Africa and Asia; there are 1 million in the United States. As with persons infected with HIV, carriers remain asymptomatic for many years, (Blumberg 1988).
[5] Unlike the morbidity and mortality among AIDS victims, the most serious consequences of syphilis occur in the later stages of the disease, among older individuals (Brandt 1988d).

analogous malady, with no cure or vaccine yet in sight, the prospects of eradicating AIDS are not bright. At the fifth international
AIDS conference held in Montreal in 1989, Samuel Broder, director
of the U.S. National Cancer Institute, declared that AIDS is a chronic
disease and that cancer is the appropriate analogue (quoted in Fee
& Fox 1992:5).

For the historian Daniel Fox and the public health analyst
Ronald Bayer, the overarching reality of AIDS is how society is being
forced to cope with it. "A decade after AIDS emerged in the United
States," Fox (1992:125) says, "most of the people who made health
policy perceived it as a stage, at present the end stage, of a chronic
disease that was spreading most rapidly among the disadvantaged,
especially among blacks and Hispanics." For Bayer (1991a), on the
other hand, it is premature to speak of AIDS itself as a chronic
disease, although "HIV infection will increasingly require the long-
term clinical management associated with such conditions" (87).

Finally, for the National Research Council's panel evaluating
the social impact of AIDS in the United States, the AIDS epidemic
differs from other epidemics in one specific way. It is not, like many
historical epidemics, "an invasion of morbidity and mortality that
rapidly sweeps through a population. It comes and will stay for
years, not only in the population, but in the individual people
infected, and its presence will often be known to them and to others
long before they suffer the disabling, lethal effects." Moreover, it is
possible to estimate the numbers of people who will be infected
years from now. "Thus," the panel concludes, "Americans must
think about this epidemic for many years into the future" (Jonsen
& Stryker 1993: 3).

AIDS and the Public

Fear of contagion: AIDS and other epidemics

Public fear reactions to epidemic disease show a remarkable
pattern of consistency from past to present. Rosenberg (1988b;
1990) notes that laypeople have always tended to be more fearful
than physicians about the dangers of interpersonal contagion; it is
a fear that antedates the germ theory. For the public, epidemic
disease has, by definition, been synonymous with the idea of
transmissibility from person to person through casual contact. In
the United States, for example, during the yellow fever and cholera
epidemics in the late eighteenth and early nineteenth centuries,
laypersons tended to reject the reassurances of medical authorities

that the diseases were not interpersonally contagious.

AIDS provides the most recent example of the phenomenon of public rejection of medical reassurances. Despite repeated announcements by scientists and medical experts that HIV infection cannot be acquired through casual contact, many people are not convinced, a fact that has serious social implications.

Brandt (1988d) adds syphilis to the catalogue of epidemic diseases that have shaped a deep-rooted and still latent fear of infection. Indeed, during the last decade of the nineteenth century and the beginning of the twentieth century, doctors as well as laypeople assumed it could be casually transmitted. But Brandt advances a different theory concerning the contemporary wariness of the public to accept the considerable scientific evidence that AIDS cannot be caught in this fashion—namely, that public health and medical authorities have not provided categorical assurances. Public misunderstanding of the nature of risk is a major contributing factor to this misperception of the danger of contagion. Americans are relatively unsophisticated in assessing relative risk, lacking the tolerance of a measure of uncertainty that is central to understanding what the concept of risk entails. When epidemiologists link the incidence of AIDS to the number of sexual contacts, Rosenberg points out, they are referring to a likelihood rather than to a certainty. Nelkin and Hilgartner (1986) cite the literature on the psychology of risk, which documents the fact that people are most fearful when the consequences of action are seen as irreversible or devastating, even if the possibility of incurring them is remote. Risks that have delayed effects are particularly frightening, which is the case with AIDS.[6] For the sociologists Perrow and Guillén (1990), what makes the AIDS epidemic strikingly different from others is the nature of the fear it inspires—a fear of unsuspected transmission and of being associated with stigmatized people such as homosexuals and intravenous drug users.

Further evidence that fear of contagion is often irrational is shown by the different perceptions the public has of different diseases. Blumberg (1988) refers to the ironic consequences of a fear gap in the case of reactions to the hepatitis B virus. Dentists were particularly vulnerable to infection with the virus (which is highly infectious) because they did not use gloves in their practice—which

---

[6] For an illustration of the problem of public perception of the risk of AIDS, see Nelkin and Hilgartner (1986). For a discussion of the fear of AIDS among physicians, see Chapter 3.

exposed them to contaminated blood. Despite this significant danger, neither the available vaccine against hepatitis B nor the practice of using rubber gloves was widely accepted. Yet when the AIDS epidemic began, the dental profession was very concerned, although it was subsequently shown that the risk of infection through dental procedures is negligible. "Despite this low risk," Blumberg remarks, "dentists are now using gloves and masks, which has the secondary and more important effect of protecting them from HBV [hepatitis B virus]. Providence works in strange ways" (409).[7]

The role of the press in shaping public reactions

No allusion to the public's fear reactions can fail to mention the role of the press and the media in shaping them. Until recently, press coverage of the epidemic in particular has been criticized as dilatory, erratic, and sensational from the very beginning. Social scientists and journalists have commented extensively on this problem. Nelkin and Hilgartner (1986), for example, point out that press coverage, especially in the early years of the epidemic, conveyed images of imminent doom. Some have held the press responsible for biased reporting that ignored the predicament of homosexuals and for excessive concern with the perception of threat held by mainstream, white, middle-class America.[8]

Sandra Panem (1988) analyzed in detail the early role of the press in contributing to public misperceptions of the threat of AIDS.

---

[7] Additional insight into the role of perception of disease in public reactions is provided by Foege (1988), who points out that the decision maker's and the public's perception of risk differs depending on whether the same disease is epidemic or endemic. He cites smallpox as an example. Smallpox was endemic in the state of Bihar in India twenty-five years ago, causing many deaths. Despite its toll, the disease did not cause panic; it was accepted and explained fatalistically. At the same time, smallpox would strike in certain regions of Africa only periodically, when it would cause panic and extensive social disruption.

[8] See James Kinsella, *Covering the Plague: AIDS and the American Media* (1990). For a discussion of the early role of the media in covering the epidemic, see Randy Shilts, *And the Band Played On: Politics, People and the AIDS Epidemic* (1987). For a different critique, see Michael Fumento, *The Myth of Heterosexual AIDS* (1990). For a review of television coverage of AIDS and its hesitancy and ambivalence in dealing with its homosexual aspects, see Cook and Colby (1992). Everett M. Rogers et al. (1991) analyze the ways in which the media have helped set the national AIDS agenda.

The press tends to support misperceived notions about the disease (such as casual transmission) that contributed to discriminatory behavior. Press coverage tended to focus on human interest stories. But Panem also refers to the press's difficulty in obtaining accurate and balanced information from the health establishment and the consequent inevitability of distortion through simplification of complex technical information. A further problem was that of identifying experts and the fact that oft-quoted media stars tend to be sought out and to achieve superstar status in the media. When expert opinion contradicts the government's official position, the result is public skepticism and confusion. Not all physicians are trained or knowledgeable about epidemiology and public health, yet the public may assume that they are all experts in all facets of the topic of AIDS. Ultimately, of course, the star status of the individuals the press listens to and quotes becomes a paramount influence in shaping the public's grasp of a major event such as AIDS.[9]

Press and television coverage at the end of the first decade of the U.S. epidemic was greatly improved in abundance, accuracy, and depth as more reports and educational materials became available from government agencies and private organizations. Nonetheless, popular misconceptions of how HIV infection is acquired still exist.

By the beginning of the second decade of AIDS, a shift in public perceptions of the American epidemic seems to have occurred. Although coverage by the media—by broadcast news reports, by hour-long TV documentaries, and by the daily press—has been generally good, public reaction has been generally passive. AIDS may be losing its power to horrify; weariness and disbelief have set in. David E. Rogers (1992:522) remarks on this numbing process: "Americans have been saturated with AIDS statistics." The result is that "they react to AIDS as they react to the homeless in our large cities—the figures are noted but fail to register in ways that evoke meaningful response. The human face of AIDS, the relentlessly progressive physical wasting and debility, the difficult-to-control pain, the emotional devastation visited upon the patients, friends and family, has faded in the blizzard of huge numbers."

Scapegoating throughout history

History shows that fear of epidemic disease, whether irratio-

---

[9] For a discussions of the role of the press in forming public conceptions of AIDS, see Rogers et al.(1991) and Chapter 9 of Panem (1988).

nal or justified, has another face. Reactions to pandemics and epidemics by frightened individuals and groups have consistently shown a pattern of assigning blame for the outbreaks to certain specific segments of society (Swenson 1988). Risse (1988:57) describes the phenomenon succinctly: "in the face of epidemic disease mankind has never reacted kindly." In an attempt to achieve distance from calamity, the human tendency has been to blame others, principally the marginal elements of communities: the poor and the alien by culture, religion, or life-style. Thus, epidemics have historically provided convenient pretexts for articulating prevailing prejudices against despised members of society, who became scapegoats.

The major targets of prejudice during the Black Death were Jews, the poor, and homosexuals (Simpson 1988). Anti-Semitism reappeared during the plague in the seventeenth century, but the poor and travelers from other plague-stricken cities were also blamed. Cholera also stigmatized Jews in the fourteenth century. In recent times, targets of scapegoating have been the poor, immigrants (the Irish principally), and Roman Catholics. During the polio epidemic of 1916, it was Italian immigrants who were blamed as carriers of the disease in Brooklyn, as were Jews and Poles in the Lower East Side of New York City (Risse 1988).[10]

The influenza epidemic called forth a different form of stereotyping which Simpson (1988) terms *international political chauvinism*, that is, stamping the disease with another national identity. The French called the epidemic "the plague of the Spanish Lady," whereas the English labeled it "the French disease." Today we characterize some strains as "Mao flu" or "Asian flu." But the disease that has epitomized this tendency throughout history is syphilis, variously called the French pox and the Spanish, Portuguese, Italian, Neapolitan, Burgundian, German, and Polish disease (Sabatier et al. 1988; Simpson 1988; Swenson 1988).

Another manifestation of the "blaming others" syndrome has been an outgrowth of the religious interpretation of disease. As Rosenberg (1988b) notes, during most previous centuries epidemic

---

[10] Later episodes of polio outbreaks during the 1950s aroused a different reaction: widespread sympathy for its victims, particularly children. Under the leadership of the National Foundation for Infantile Paralysis, a voluntary association, this outpouring of sympathy was institutionalized in the immensely successful March of Dimes, a yearly fund-raising event that provided the funds for research on the polio vaccine (Sills 1957).

disease was perceived in "moral and transcendent" terms. Lacking knowledge about the etiology of epidemics, society has interpreted these events in religious terms—as divine punishments for moral transgression. Disease was seen as punishment for sinners and therefore a result of their own actions. As Rosenberg writes, "The desire to explain sickness and death in terms of volition—of acts done or left undone—is ancient and powerful" (27).

The plagues of the Middle Ages were seen as divine visitations upon the victims as well as the fault of pariah groups (Keniston 1990). Leprosy,[11] "the most ancient of plagues," was widespread in the Middle Ages. An endemic rather than an epidemic disease, it was linked to sexual promiscuity in medieval society and became a metaphor for moral turpitude and excessive lust (Musto 1988:70–71). Smallpox was once confused with syphilis and it thus inherited its moral stigma. It was not until the nineteenth century that the two diseases were distinguished medically, but the conceptual connection persisted (Nelkin & Gilman 1988). Cholera was conceived in religious terms as a punishment for a sinful society at large (Simpson 1988). Tuberculosis was often seen as the fault of the consumptive (Musto 1988). Syphilis, which associated death with sexual activity, is often referred to as the prime example of the embodiment of moral censure by the public at large. But it was not always so. Kenneth M. Ludmerer (1989), a physician and historian of medicine at Washington University in St. Louis, points out that in times when attitudes toward sex outside marriage have been liberal, especially among the upper classes, syphilis has been rampant, and not censured. During the Renaissance, for example, particularly among the nobility, when extramarital affairs were fashionable, and during the next two and a half centuries, it was not considered shameful to have contracted the disease. Emperors, kings, noblemen, churchmen, scholars, and poets are said to have spoken openly of their disease. During the eighteenth century, a time of great sexual licentiousness, Ludmerer reports, syphilis was almost a badge of distinction. The symbols of the era were Don Juan and Casanova. Attitudes changed with the rise of the middle class with its bourgeois values that emphasized the sanctity of the family and condemned licentiousness.

By the nineteenth century, condemnation of syphilis had become dominant in Western society. Syphilis was perceived as a

---

[11] Leprosy, caused by a bacillus, was until modern times thought to be highly contagious through casual contact (Musto 1988).

symbol of illicit promiscuity, a threat to the Victorian system of social norms, and a violation of the sanctity of marriage and the family. It was a disease of the so-called guilty (Fee 1988). During the first decades of the twentieth century, distinctions were drawn between the guilty—that is, erring husbands—and innocent victims—that is, their wives and children (Rosenberg 1988b). During the wave of immigration from the end of the nineteenth to the first decade of the twentieth centuries, the targets of opprobrium were immigrants and prostitutes.

During World War I, Army propaganda directed at soldiers carried the message that "a German bullet is cleaner than a whore" (Brandt 1988a:368). Voluntary associations such as the Social Hygiene Association, which equated venereal disease with immorality, advocated sexual abstinence and tried to close brothels and taverns. During the 1930s in Baltimore, where rates of syphilis were high, the disease was seen as a problem specifically among blacks, who were linked with promiscuous behavior (Fee 1988). Again, when, despite the availability of antibiotics, syphilis infection spiraled again during the 1960s, this was attributed to "the three 'p's', permissiveness, promiscuity and the pill" (Brandt 1988d: 379).

The blaming syndrome and AIDS discrimination

The AIDS pandemic has repeated the pattern of scapegoating demonstrated in the past. Scapegoating is worldwide, as Jonathan Mann repeated in many public speeches, press interviews, and policy statements of the Global Programme on AIDS, characterizing it as an "epidemic" in itself. As Sapolsky (1990) notes, the fear of AIDS divides communities everywhere as subgroups have sought safety in isolation from one another. In the United States, AIDS has also provided ample opportunity to cast blame (Swenson 1988).

When the spectrum of symptoms of HIV infection was first identified as a new disease, medical authorities called it GRID (gay-related immunodeficiency disease), a fact that has had implications for the official response to AIDS. The death from AIDS of the movie actor Rock Hudson in 1986 dramatized the identification of AIDS in the public mind as a disease of homosexuals (Treichler 1988). The Centers for Disease Control's identification in 1981 and 1982 of other risk groups such as Haitians, intravenous drug users, hemophiliacs, blacks, and Hispanics reinforced a popular perception of these groups as the root causes of AIDS (Porter 1989; Treichler 1988). This classification helped promote a discriminatory view of the disease and, as Treichler remarks, has contributed to the perception that the major risk factor in acquiring the disease is membership in a particular group rather than individual behavior. As Porter points out, when the public came to see Haitian immigrants as carriers, they became targets of backlash in major cities—against store owners, domestics, and schoolchildren.

The public's inherent desire to distance itself from groups viewed as disease carriers was reinforced in the early years of the epidemic by an unfortunate remark Margaret Heckler—then the secretary of health, education, and welfare, made at the International conference on AIDS in Atlanta in 1985. She stressed the urgent need to "conquer AIDS . . . before it affects the heterosexual population and threatens the health of our general population." The statement was widely interpreted by homosexuals and blacks as hostile (quoted in Dalton 1990:253).

Irrational fear of AIDS has aroused the same feelings of hostility towards victims of the disease that have characterized other epidemics. Although, happily, violent episodes have been relatively rare, parents have made many attempts to exclude children infected with AIDS from attending public schools.[12] AIDS victims have faced, and are still facing, discrimination in the workplace, restaurants, apartment buildings, housing,[13] hospitals, and doctors' offices (Gray 1989; Kass 1987; Nelkin & Hilgartner 1986).

A survey by the American Civil Liberties Union AIDS Project (Hunter 1990), reviewing 13,000 reported cases of discrimination, concludes that bias against people with AIDS, expressed in acts of discrimination, have been increasing despite increased knowledge about how the disease is transmitted. Based on questionnaires sent to 600 organizations, including state and city human rights com-

---

[12] Poirier (1988) reports two such instances, that is, the torching of the home of three AIDS-infected hemophiliac boys in Arcadia, Florida, and a similar attack on a house in London. Among the more famous recent cases is that of Ryan White, a 12-year-old hemophiliac infected through a blood transfusion who became the target of a community effort to ban him from attending classes. White became an activist for tolerance and understanding of AIDS victims, achieving national fame before he died of AIDS at the age of 18. For a discussion of the legal aspects of the White case, see Kass (1987).

[13] One example of housing discrimination was reported in the *New York Times* (March 14, 1988:A14). The Texas Association of Realtors, meeting in Houston, told its members that occupancy by an AIDS patient could be viewed by prospective buyers as a defect of the house, much like a bad roof or the presence of radon gas. Therefore, agents were urged to disclose this information to prospective buyers to avoid lawsuits.

missions, legal aid services, and AIDS service organizations, the report indicates that discrimination has increased faster than the number of AIDS cases during the same period (1984–1988). A surprising finding is that about 30 percent of the cases of discrimination were not against those already infected, but against those perceived to be at risk for HIV infection—as well as against individuals who care for AIDS patients. The most frequent site of discrimination (37 percent) is the workplace—although no instances of transmission have been documented in this setting (outside of health care settings). Employees have been dismissed in several states once their HIV status became known to employers. Other instances of discrimination documented by the report are in housing, in nursing homes, and in other health care settings (where physicians and nurses and dentists refused treatment of persons with AIDS); and against persons applying for insurance.[14]

AIDS as volition: Moralistic censure

Public perceptions of AIDS duplicate conceptions of illness that have prevailed in other epidemics—namely that the disease is the fault of the afflicted. In a preface to an interdisciplinary collection of essays on the AIDS epidemic, the editor, Padraig O'Malley (1989:5), observed that AIDS seems to satisfy "our predilection for punitive notions of disease." The snide joke labeling AIDS as WOGS—the "Wrath of God Syndrome"—is an example of a popular denigration.

AIDS has also aroused the same moralistic condemnation that identified the outbreaks of syphilis at the end of the nineteenth and the first two decades of the twentieth century. Indeed, as Brandt (1988c:152) observes, "it is almost impossible to watch the AIDS epidemic without a sense of *déjà vu*." The parallels are striking: "a fatal disease without the promise of a magic bullet" on the horizon and one that is fraught with conflicts concerning the risks of sexuality and the nature of social responsibility. Friedland (1990), describing some reactions to patients in a large medical center,

---

[14] The problem of discrimination resulting from the AIDS epidemic has spawned an increasingly voluminous literature detailing how the law has dealt with many manifestations of discrimination. An early compendium is *AIDS and the Law*, edited by Harlan L. Dalton et al. (1989). A review of 149 cases of discrimination is included in an article by Lawrence O. Gostin (1992). A third useful guide for the general reader is *Living with AIDS* (1987), a pamphlet published by the Lambda Legal Defense and Education Fund.

refers to AIDS being seen as a dirty disease; for many, it remains a disease of illicit intimacy.

As was the case with syphilis, the same distinctions prevail in the public mind between "innocent" victims and the "guilty," the media perpetuate this dichotomy. Press and television "human interest" stories have stressed the need for compassion for the accidental recipients (usually portrayed as middle class) of contaminated blood transfusions received during hospital stays for illnesses unrelated to AIDS; for hemophiliacs who have received transfusions of an AIDS-infected clotting factor; for children born to infected mothers; and for health care workers infected through needle sticks. By inference, innuendo, or the statements of a minority of outspoken critics, reported in the press—particularly in the early stage of the AIDS epidemic—the "guilty" have been the homosexuals, drug addicts, immigrants suspected of bisexual behavior, the promiscuous poor in ghetto areas, prostitutes, and the homeless. As Nelkin and Gilman (1988) point out, "the rhetoric of blame" (363) ignores the fact that certain kinds of behavior (homosexuality) "may not be entirely voluntary" (371).[15]

The concept of blame has been reinforced by statements articulated by some religious leaders and political conservatives. Echoing the Papal Bull of 1348 which described the Black Death as "the pestilence with which God is afflicting the Christian people" are such comments by contemporary conservatives as "AIDS is the wrath of God upon homosexuals" (Altman 1986:66–67). The conservative columnist William F. Buckley publicly advocated tattooing all HIV-positive individuals on their buttocks and isolating them from society (Ron & Rogers 1990:111).[16] These sentiments have been echoed by the magazine *Commentary*, whose editor, Norman Podhoretz, criticized crash programs to develop an AIDS vaccine as providing covert sanction for homosexuality (Richards 1988).

Another political expression of this stance is the opposition of Senator Jesse Helms, Republican of North Carolina, to a bill approved by the Senate on May 17, 1990, granting emergency relief

---

[15] Friedland (1990:136) sees drug addiction in this light. "It is not a matter of chance," he points out, "that rates of intravenous drug use are highest among poor minorities in the inner city." Not the victims of addiction, Friedland asserts, but the societal conditions that breed this type of behavior are to blame: unemployment, poverty, racism, and hopelessness.

[16] The suggestion prompted Gray (1989:234) to label it "a modern-day version of the leper's bell"; it also reminded Ron and Rogers (1990:111) of "leper colonies of the past."

to cities and states hardest hit by the epidemic. Objecting to the defeat of amendments that would have made it a criminal offense for prostitutes, HIV-positive individuals, and drug addicts to donate blood to blood banks, Helms stated that without these provisions, the bill treated homosexual sex as a normal part of one's life-style, a "perverted, illegal, and immoral activity that must be stopped in order to end the AIDS epidemic." He labeled the measure a "weapon" for the "deterioration if not the destruction of America's Judeo-Christian value system" (*New York Times*, May 17, 1990:B10). A review of public opinion surveys by two Harvard sociologists reported on a high level of intolerance and willingness to discriminate against people afflicted with AIDS, coupled with a high level of fear and concern (Blendon & Donelan 1990).

Ronald Bayer has predicted that the "ghettoization of HIV transmission" (1989:241) will undoubtedly increase racism and disgust for the underclass. Although a joint CBS/*New York Times* survey subsequently found that 85 percent of the public showed "a lot of" or "some" sympathy towards PWAs, only 39 percent of the respondents said that they had "a lot of sympathy" for PWAs who became infected through homosexual encounters and only 30 per cent said they had sympathy for people who share needles during drug injections. Moreover, 57 percent said that the United States should keep people who test positive from entering the country to live here permanently and 49 percent said the country should keep infected tourists out of the country (*New York Times*, June 18, 1991:C3)

Public opinion polls conducted since 1987 (Singer 1991; 1993) provide overviews of public opinion trends regarding AIDS victims over the years. More than two-fifths of the respondents to Roper polls during these years saw AIDS as a punishment for the decline of moral standards. A May 1991 Gallup poll showed a slight decline in this negative response and more than four out of five respondents expressed "a lot" or "some" sympathy for PWAs—but the favorable response dropped dramatically if the disease was described as being a result of homosexual activity (39 percent) or from sharing needles while taking illegal drugs (30 percent).

Paranoia about AIDS

The phenomenon of blaming the victim is not a practice limited to white Americans. Some leaders of the black community have labeled AIDS a "gay white man's disease," when in fact twice as many blacks and Hispanics, as would have been expected by their numbers, are afflicted with the disease. And according to Harlon Dalton, a professor at Yale Law School and a member of the National Commission on AIDS, black hostility against gays is a barrier the black community must overcome in making progress against the epidemic. Indeed, he notes that "more than once I have heard of black parents readily volunteering, so as to forestall more embarrassing speculation, that their HIV infected children are addicts" (Dalton 1990:245). The black community's slow response to the need to fight AIDS, Dalton says, has been this reluctance to being associated with what is perceived as an immoral gay disease. Moreover, blacks have been outraged by many assertions concerning the African origins of AIDS, since "we understand in our bones that with origin comes blame." In addition, the singling out of Haitians as a risk group by the Centers for Disease Control "simply confirmed our worst fears" (1990:244).

Misperceptions and fear of AIDS have spawned a bizarre reaction among some members of the black community. A *New York Times* editorial, "The AIDS 'Plot against Blacks'" (May 12, 1992:A22) cited several surveys that revealed paranoid reactions to AIDS. One survey of black church members revealed that 35 percent of the respondents believed that AIDS was a form of black genocide; a CBS/*New York Times* survey in 1990 found that one in ten blacks believed that the AIDS virus had been "deliberately created in a laboratory in order to infect black people" and an additional two in ten thought that this might be so; and a Gallup/*Newsweek* poll in March 1992 showed similar results. The *Times* editorial also reported a black health worker's testimony before the National Commission on AIDS revealing the belief that AIDS is a "man-made" disease; that some blacks believe that the drug AZT is a plot to poison them; that campaigns urging condom use to prevent HIV infection are a scheme to reduce the number of black babies; and that the distribution of clean needles to black drug addicts is a plot to encourage drug use. These fears, fueled by knowledge of the infamous 1932–72 Tuskegee syphilis study (in which blacks were denied treatment in order to test the natural course of syphilis and were told year after year that they were actually being treated) has reduced African-American participation in clinical trials of new drugs, according to the report of the National Commission on AIDS.

Bias breeds intolerance and discrimination. The growing evidence of this fact prompted the National Commission on AIDS in December 1989 to urge the White House to formulate a statement on the need to dispense care to AIDS victims without discrimination.

Responding to this call, President Bush issued a statement, widely reported in the media, about the need for understanding and compassion without assigning blame toward those suffering from AIDS:

> For those who are living with HIV and AIDS, our response is clear: They deserve our compassion . . . Once disease strikes—we don't blame those who are suffering. We don't spurn the accident victim who didn't wear a seatbelt. We don't reject the cancer patient who didn't quit smoking. We try to love them and care for them and comfort them. We do not fire them, or evict them, or cancel their insurance (quoted in National Commission on AIDS 1990a:1).

Illness as individual responsibility

This discussion of the classic phenomenon of "blaming the victim" of disease is not complete without reference to its broader and uniquely contemporary cultural context. Nelkin and Hilgartner, writing in 1986, noted a contributing trend—namely, the increasing emphasis on preventive medicine and on the role of individual responsibility in maintaining health over the last decade. They called attention to the conclusion of a Surgeon General's report of 1979 entitled *Healthy People: The Surgeon General's Report on Health Promotion and Disease Prevention*, which became a "manifesto" of the role of life-style in avoiding disease. Describing the features of what amounts to a contemporary social movement, the report points out that the tendency to place blame on individual behavior is a "ubiquitous" theme in a variety of diseases, including cancer.[17] One outstanding example of its acceptance is the (at least partial) success in reducing cigarette smoking among the public to avoid cancer. The increasing drumbeat of advertisements in the media for foods said to be healthier, the success of health newslet-

---

[17] The critic Susan Sontag is widely quoted in the literature on AIDS for her thesis that certain serious, life-threatening illnesses, like tuberculosis and cancer, and more recently, AIDS, have unfortunately become "metaphorized." That is, they have acquired nonmedical overtones of symbolism and are thus seen as markers of character flaws rather than as outcomes of biological processes. Associated with weakness, moral corruption, and pollution, AIDS itself has in her view become a stigma, born of moralistic judgment. See her *Illness as Metaphor* (1978) and *AIDS and Its Metaphors* (1988).

ters sponsored by major universities, and the proliferation of health programs on public television all attest to the general notion that Americans increasingly accept personal responsibility for their health. The acceptance of personal responsibility for harmful behavior is not a moral triumph but rather implies the notion of achieving control over disease.

6

Governmental Responses

A distinguishing characteristic of epidemics is that they generate a sharp sense of crisis and an immediate demand for decisive and visible national and community action. Historians see this pattern of response as replete with relevant parallels and implications for the responses to AIDS.

Historical precedents for the control of epidemic disease

Since the fourteenth century, quarantine has been the most common organized response of the authorities responsible for protecting the health of the public. But quarantine, according to Musto (1988) and Brandt (1988c), has traditionally been largely an expression of public fears about the outsider or about socially marginal groups. It has been more a response to popular demands to create boundaries between the sick urban masses and the respectable segments of mainstream society than it has been an effective means of controlling disease. Rosenberg (1990) and Slack (1988) also see quarantine as primarily a rationale for the social control of outgroups rather than as a method of combating contagion. Lepers were segregated in the Middle Ages; quarantine measures in medieval Italy during the bubonic plague were part of a campaign against beggars and prostitutes.[1] In the seventeenth century, plague quarantine hospitals (*lazarettos*) were established, and violators of public health regulations were sometimes executed (Risse 1988).

---

[1] For a detailed description of public health measures used during the bubonic plague epidemics in medieval Europe, see Slack (1988).

During the nineteenth century cholera epidemic, blanket quarantine measures were taken in New York to bar all passengers and goods from Asia and Africa in an attempt to stem the spread of the disease to the United States. Later, when the disease struck the city itself, individuals suspected of being infected were taken to makeshift hospitals for observation. Each admission was classified as "temperate" or "intemperate" or "uncertain" (Risse 1988:45). However, the response to the recurrent cholera epidemics in the United States and England also had positive results. Many of our current public health laws were enacted during the mid-nineteenth century and are still in effect. Local boards of health were established, cholera hospitals were founded, food and drug control measures were initiated, slum clearance was undertaken, and housing and care for the destitute were provided (Swenson 1988).

Quarantine measures were again invoked in combating yellow fever, despite the fact that the disease is not contagious from one person to another (Musto 1988). During the pre-World War II polio epidemics in the United States, quarantine efforts to isolate victims resulted in house-to-house searches, the separation of sick children from their parents, and the placarding of children in their homes for two weeks. A ban on travel outside New York City was enforced, while surrounding summer resort towns on Long Island imposed their own restrictions against vacationing New Yorkers (Risse 1988).

Tuberculosis, whose high death rates made it one of the most feared diseases,[2] led to measures imposing mandatory treatment for "careless consumptives." U.S. immigration laws of the early twentieth century carried the notion of quarantine one step further towards racial discrimination, limiting the influx of immigrants who were seen as carriers of disease (Musto 1988).[3]

---

[2] Rosenberg (1990) reports that one of the defining characteristics of epidemics is that they generate public pressure for a decisive and visible community response. Yet tuberculosis, despite the fact that in the nineteenth century its toll was higher than yellow fever or cholera, did not elicit the sense of crisis that these other epidemics aroused.

[3] Musto (1988) notes that when drug addiction was viewed as a contagion, it became another basis for discrimination against immigrants: opium smoking was linked to the Chinese, heroin was associated with European immigrants, cocaine with South Americans, hashish with Africans. Fear of these despised minorities as carriers of drug addiction led to the restrictive immigration laws of the 1920s. In the 1960s, when there was a sudden increase in drug addiction, being an addict could make a person subject to involuntary confinement for therapeutic purposes. A Supreme Court decision

The most directly relevant antecedents to the organized official response to epidemic disease are the public health interventions undertaken at the beginning of the twentieth century to prevent the spread of venereal infection. It was in 1918, as Brandt (1988c) points out, that initiatives for disease reporting, screening, testing, and isolation were taken. Even though it was known that syphilis could not be spread by casual contact, compulsory screening of food handlers and barbers was mandated by some municipalities.[4] But the most extreme public health measures were directed against prostitutes during World War I. Gostin (1986), a specialist in health law, reports that tens of thousands of prostitutes were quarantined as real or suspected carriers of venereal disease.[5] Brandt (1988d) describes this crackdown as a concerted attack on civil liberties in the name of public health.[6] Nonetheless, these measures had no visible impact on venereal disease rates. In the 1920s and 1940s, Public Health Service health statistics were analyzed by race: syphilis, for example, was identified as a problem of the black population (Fee 1988). During World War II, in contrast to the earlier war, the emphasis was on educational campaigns, for the military had now recognized that modifying sexual behavior is the most effective means of controlling the spread of infection.

In 1936, under the leadership of Surgeon General Thomas Parran, a campaign was launched to disassociate syphilis from moral condemnation by the public at large and to develop programs to combat the disease. In 1938, the National Venereal Disease Control Act established diagnostic laboratories and clinics for voluntary testing. In addition, the Wassermann test was offered to the public for premarital screening, first on a voluntary basis (Fee 1988:129).

---

declared that a state was empowered to establish a program of compulsory treatment for narcotic addicts and that "such a program ... might require periods of involuntary confinement." Justice William O. Douglas, in a concurring opinion, added that confinement might be justified "for the good of society" (quoted in Musto 1988:79).

[4] Brandt (1988d) reports that during World War I the U.S. Navy removed doorknobs from its battleships, claiming they were a source of syphilis infection.

[5] Brandt (1988c) reports the figure of more than 20,000 women quarantined through federally funded action and thousands more incarcerated through local programs.

[6] Gostin also discusses how in some cases the power of quarantine was misused, for example, without proof that a prostitute was even infectious.

By 1945, all the states had made premarital screening for syphilis mandatory before obtaining a marriage license. However, compulsory premarital screening proved ineffective as a way of identifying new cases. The problem was that the test yielded false-positive results: about a quarter of the individuals who tested positive were actually not infected. Nevertheless, as Brandt (1988d:379) reports, these individuals "often underwent toxic treatments on the assumption that the tests were correct." More-over, some managed to avoid being tested. As a result, by the early 1980s a number of states repealed their mandatory screening laws. During World War II, nonpunitive measures by the military, com-bined with penicillin, proved highly successful. Brandt attributes the steep rise in rates of syphilis during the 1960s, noted earlier, to a decrease in public funding for coordinated efforts of this kind as much as to a loosening of standards of sexual behavior.[7]

Controlling the spread of AIDS

The task of controlling the AIDS epidemic—that is, of moni-toring its dimensions, of identifying the various categories of its victims, of containing its propagation to the general public, of alerting the public to its dangers, and of seeking to control the behavior that causes it to spread—is a uniquely intricate one. As a report of the Institute of Medicine states:

> If a panel of public health experts, lawyers, economists, and sociologists had been asked a decade ago to imag-ine a public health problem that would encompass the most difficult policy issues of the day, they could not have done better than to predict the appearance of AIDS (Institute of Medicine 1986b:132).

Quite apart from the problems intrinsic to the complicated nature of the disease is the social context in which it is occurring— a context of greater sensitivity to civil rights in general and the rights of minorities in particular; a climate of greater tolerance for uncon-ventional life styles and widespread sexual permissiveness than at any previous period in American history; and a period of increasing concern with ethical considerations involving individual rights in

---

[7] One extreme contemporary example of a government's response to the threat of AIDS is that of the Ministry of Public Health of Thailand, which reportedly drafted a law on AIDS which in effect made criminals of individuals infected with HIV (*The Economist*, September 15, 1990).

illness and death. Added to these long-range concerns and issues are the short-term dynamics of rival political philosophies and the limitations of an economy geared to social spending reductions and faced with massive costs in AIDS health care and research. More specifically, the AIDS crisis has created policy conflicts, ethical and legal dilemmas, and contradictions on various levels of government concerning the enforcement of prevention programs.

Finally, the official response to AIDS has raised fundamental philosophical issues concerning the government's obligation to protect the health of the public at large and, in turn, concerning the responsibility of individuals for spreading the disease through risky behavior. It has raised the issue of the civil rights of individuals—for example, the rights to privacy and to confidentiality—versus what some perceive as the public's right to protect itself against the danger of infection.

Policy conflicts concerning the use of drugs

The U.S AIDS epidemic has fostered a major clash of policy objectives between the war on drugs and the war on AIDS. This conflict stems from proposals to provide clean needles to drug addicts as a means of slowing the spread of HIV infection among intravenous drug users. Critics of the proposals, of course, maintain that such programs would increase drug use, but there are both advocates and opponents in many public agencies as well as outside the government (Fox et al. 1990).

The enforcement of antidrug policies and the creation of needle exchange programs are in direct conflict. For June Osborn (1990), exchange programs—although not lasting solutions to the problem of HIV infection through drug use—have merit if they represent the sole option for persons driven by their addiction into sharing contaminated needles. The controlled exchange of clean for dirty needles in areas of high infection may be a logical and important stopgap measure for cities like New York, where more than 200,000 persons are estimated to be addicted to intravenous heroin, of whom only 40,000 can be accommodated by drug detoxification programs.[8] (Of these 200,000, half are believed to be HIV-infected.)

---

[8]Osborn (1990) points out that needle exchange programs have been established in many European cities. While final results concerning the reduction of HIV infection are not known, there has not been any suggestion of increased drug use as a result.

Osborn reports that the commissioners of health for New York City and New York State took opposite positions on the proposal to launch a trial needle exchange program. An indictment of needle exchanging was articulated by Harlon Dalton, who in addition to being a law professor and a black, is also a member of the National Commission on AIDS. He voiced the sentiments of the black community with these rhetorical questions:

> You say that making drug use safer . . . won't make it more attractive to our children or our neighbors' children? But what if you are wrong? What if as a result we have even more addicts to contend with ? . . . Why do you offer addicts free needles but not free health care? . . . Why not provide immediate treatment for every addict who wants it? (Dalton 1990:251).

Testing and screening issues

The presence of infection with the AIDS virus can only be determined by serological tests showing the presence of antibodies to HIV in the blood. The use of this basic scientific tool has spawned a host of controversies, ethical conflicts, and legal problems.

Testing the blood of individuals who show symptoms that are suggestive of AIDS—with their consent and as part of a diagnostic workup in doctors' offices, hospitals, and clinics—has not posed ethical problems (Levine & Bayer 1989). At issue, however, is the mandatory testing of individuals without symptoms. This program has been the subject of intense critical scrutiny by public health experts, AIDS activists, and ethicists. The concern is that not only individuals with AIDS but also those who are HIV positive face the possibility of discrimination in obtaining or maintaining health insurance, in housing, in employment, in finding physicians to treat them, and, of course in maintaining close social relationships with others.

Mandatory testing and screening of populations raises the quandary posed by the need to balance protecting the public at large from disease and protecting individual freedom, a civil right. A traditional public health strategy has been to control infectious diseases by identifying carriers: in the past, actions of this kind have been preludes to quarantine.

During the first decade of the AIDS epidemic, public demands for mandatory testing and screening came from school boards, pressured by parents anxious about the safety of their children in school, from hospital admission departments, from unions, from employers, and from prison authorities. They also came from state governments. In fact, by 1987 many states had made proposals for premarital screening. (Two states, Illinois and Louisiana, passed statutes mandating this measure but renounced the effort within the year as largely unenforceable and not worth the attempt.) Right-wing political groups, such as the one headed by Lyndon La Rouche in California, in a referendum known as Proposition 64, called for mandatory universal screening for the purpose of identifying carriers of the disease and of isolating them. Opposed by the entire public health community, by physicians, and by the press, the proposition was defeated by the electorate in 1988 (Fox et al. 1990). The federal government uses mandatory testing and screening programs for military recruits, for members of the foreign service, and for immigrants (Bayer 1989).

The central ethical question that is at the heart of debates on mandatory testing and screening has been their potential for violating the individual's right to privacy—a violation that may come about with the unwarranted disclosure of information that should be treated as privileged and that can lead to various forms of discrimination and social ostracism. In both Australia and Sweden, major disagreements have arisen over provisions regarding the confidentiality of antibody tests (Altman 1988). In Australia, there has been strong public opinion support for the mandatory testing of homosexuals, immigrants, and tourists (Kirby 1990). The ethicist LeRoy Walters (1988) emphasized that the AIDS epidemic has forced the authorities to choose between controlling it and unjustly discriminating against particular social groups. There is scant justification and little responsible public support for universal antibody screening programs, he pointed out, whether voluntary or compulsory, because the blood tests that are employed are not foolproof and may produce false-positive results. Furthermore, they are very costly, since they would have to be repeated periodically.

Debates have centered on whether selective screening of two types—both voluntary and compulsory—is justified for groups such as hemophiliacs, intravenous drug users, prostitutes, patients in clinics that treat sexually transmitted diseases, military recruits and personnel, hospital patients (candidates for surgery and hemodialysis), and prisoners. This selective screening is said to be justifiable only if these programs are conducted in a context that (1) provides guarantees of confidentiality by statute, (2) guarantees against discrimination, and (3) is accompanied by counseling. "In a democratic society," Walters concluded, "the presumption should be in favor of voluntary rather than mandatory public health programs" (599). Lawrence Gostin (1987), a lawyer, voiced objections to mandatory mass screening on the grounds that even the most ambitious program ever discussed would not reveal the actual number of infected people. Ronald Bayer (1989) objected on civil libertarian grounds. For Michael Kirby (1990), an Australian jurist who is also a member of the WHO Global Commission on AIDS, the inconsistencies inherent in mandatory testing policies practiced internationally discriminate against marginalized groups. He pointed out that there are also inconsistencies in these policies. To test immigrants but not tourists is unjustifiable, since tourists may have had greater exposure to AIDS. To test prisoners without arranging for the care of the infected is pointless and irresponsible, yet in prisons around the world, compulsory testing is occurring at an increasing rate.[9]

June Osborn (1990) advances a different argument against coercive approaches to screening. She points out that mandatory testing of potential donors of blood has protected both the blood supply and donated organs and tissues, and thus has been a wise policy. However, the urge to extend this mandate to other groups in the population has been irresistible to many politicians: the political scene has been flooded with proposals to use the antibody tests to identify HIV-infected individuals. This has occurred despite almost unanimous warnings by public health experts that draconian measures of this sort are sure to drive underground the very people at risk and most in need of education and counseling. Policies of quarantine or isolation that would follow such an approach, she writes, "are no more relevant to HIV than an onslaught of cavalry would have been in the tactical landscape of Vietnam" (402).

The spectrum of opinions on the thorny issue of screening would not be complete without including a dissenting British view. Robert M. May and his Oxford biologist colleagues (1990) articulate the underlying dilemma of screening. Although they recognize the legitimate concerns for the infected individual's privacy and rights, as well as the moral obligation and need for an unambiguous legal obligation to prevent discrimination against the infected, they warn that excessive precautions have sometimes interfered with the gathering of essential data. Their concluding statement reads:

---

[9] The issue of testing individuals seeking entry into the United States has been hotly debated. In early 1991, it was asserted that the restrictions would be lifted on June 21, 1991, but subsequent developments have changed this time frame. See Chapter 4 for developments in early 1993.

Such inaccessibility of information potentially sacri-
fices the rights of invisible individuals—the HIV infections waiting downstream in time, as it were—some of
whom might be spared if we understood the epidemic
better. Conflicting concerns of this kind are as old as
humanity itself. We believe, however, that we should
stretch hard to find acceptable ways of making all data
available and of systematically acquiring new data. We
should not wait until people actually become infected
with HIV before we acknowledge their rights (May et al.
1990:100).

Ronald Bayer has articulated the fundamental social conflict
transcending individual interests in the struggle to control the
epidemic. In his book, *Private Acts, Social Consequences* (1989), Bayer
says that what makes the public health response to the threat of
AIDS so troubling for a liberal society is that the transmission of the
disease involves intimate social relationships that have in the past
been resistant to social control: sexual acts between men and
women, as well as homosexual acts and the techniques of intravenous
drug use. At the same time, the civil liberties and civil rights
movements advancing the cause of blacks, women, and homosexuals have been strengthening constitutional guarantees that limit the
state's authority over individual freedom and that protect individual
privacy. "Against this constitutional tradition and social ethos,"
Bayer writes, "AIDS has forced a confrontation with the problem of
how to respond to private acts that have critical social consequences"
(5).

The danger in confronting the AIDS threat, according to
Michael Kirby (1990), is that democratically elected governments
will succumb to public pressure for action by enacting legislation
restricting the freedom of marginal groups (such as prostitutes,
drug users, and prisoners)—groups otherwise lacking an effective
voice to defend their rights. Traditionally, societies attempt to
inculcate individual responsibility through laws that have a deterrent symbolic value. And indeed, in both the United States and
Australia, calls have been made for listing specific criminal offenses
for which, on conviction, courts may penalize the deliberate or
reckless spread of the lethal virus. Kirby warns that overenthusiasm
in enacting such laws may make some people feel better, but they
will have little impact on the spread of the epidemic. The need is to
accompany laws and policies on AIDS with protection against

discrimination—a principle repeatedly affirmed by the reports of both then-Surgeon General Koop and the presidential advisory commissions. The lessons of history in the management of syphilis are that attempts to deal with it punitively, by stigmatization and the harsh regulation of prostitutes, have been failures.[10]

The second decade of the AIDS epidemic has brought a change in the nature of the controversies surrounding screening and testing. In an article in *Health Affairs*, Bayer (1991a) traced the change in emphasis in these debates brought about by the realization that HIV infection would increasingly require the long-term clinical management associated with chronic diseases. Public health officials are now faced with a dual problem: not only must they prevent infection, but they must also provide care for the million or more Americans who are infected with the virus and require clinical supervision. As a consequence, it has become crucial to identify the infected individuals. Issues such as screening and mandatory testing that had been challenged as threats to privacy and confidentiality in the 1980s have now found new support from the very groups that had rejected them as unacceptable. The traditional public health measures of HIV antibody testing and reporting the names of infected individuals are now seen as inevitable adjuncts to providing Medicaid coverage for the early treatment of the HIV-infected in government-funded clinics. The move towards early clinical intervention, Bayer (1992:87) has subsequently pointed out, is in effect incompatible with the preservation of anonymity. The central political and ethical question of privacy, which was debated in the epidemic's first phase, "has now been joined, although not displaced, by that of equity."

Criticism of the U.S. government's response to AIDS

The chronicle of the fight against AIDS, which began more than a decade ago in the United States, has been marked from the beginning by (1) controversy over policies concerning the best methods of combating the spreading infection; (2) acrimonious accusations by patient advocate groups seeking a greater commitment of government resources in search of a cure and a vaccine, as well as drugs for therapy; and (3) conservative political pressure to

---

[10] For a detailed analysis of the failure of compulsory health measures to control syphilis epidemics, see Brandt (1988a).

shape more stringent regulations for controlling the epidemic. Much of the conservative political pressure, according to Osborn (1990), has been inspired by inappropriate analogies with past epidemics, such as plague and polio.

The problems, the dilemmas of choice involved in combating AIDS, lie in the domain of science, medicine, economics, and the law—both on the federal and state levels—as well as in agency, White House, and congressional policy decisions. The series of public health policies, regulations, activities, and legislative actions, whose sum total represents the official response to AIDS, has thus been subjected to intense scrutiny in a voluminous and growing literature.

Criticism has come from various quarters: from scientists and public health physicians critical of the various agencies involved in combating the epidemic; from lawyers specializing in public health law; from judges and other legal professionals concerned with protecting civil rights in various settings, such as housing and the workplace; from persons concerned with providing such services as medical care and access to insurance; from political scientists, sociologists, and others concerned with the dynamics of policy choices and the structure of institutions dealing with the control of epidemics; from the Institute of Medicine of the National Research Council—a private, nonprofit agency chartered by Congress to advise the government; and from within the administrations of presidents Ronald Reagan and George Bush—in the form of reports from two presidential advisory commissions that have issued evaluative studies of the nation's war against AIDS.

Nature of the criticism

The most common criticism has been that the national response to AIDS was tardy, that the Reagan administration and its agencies responsible for public health and for biomedical research were slow to recognize the implications of the onset of AIDS.

The prominent biomedical researcher Robert Gallo has responded to the specific criticism that the medical research establishment (himself included) was slow in showing interest in AIDS because it was then seen as a disease of homosexuals:

> Such thinking shows a failure to understand how scientists choose what to work on. Scientists are drawn to problems that seem capable of solution given the present state of knowledge, specifically those problems

where their own abilities and training make a personal contribution possible and address a societal need. . . To say that I failed to be interested in a disease that struck down fellow human beings because the sexual practices of some of its victims may have been different from mine is egregiously absurd (Gallo 1991:133).

The first and most trenchant published indictment of the government's response—one that aroused widespread popular interest—was a work of advocacy by the journalist Randy Shilts (1987). His book, the widely cited *And the Band Played On*, is focused principally on the period between the late 1970s and 1985a—period during which the scope of the epidemic had not become fully evident. Its central thesis is that the federal government was dilatory in responding to the evidence of the outbreak of a new disease—which it perceived as a disease of the homosexual community—a delay compounded by a lack of cooperation among health agencies.

Swenson (1988) also noted that during the early 1980s it was common to hear statements that AIDS was not a major epidemic—that is, to deny its existence. As epidemiological data began to accumulate, showing that the principal targets of the disease were not only homosexuals but drug users as well, this denial took a different form, namely, disbelief that the disease would eventually spread from these circumscribed groups to other segments of society. Public health physicians Aron Ron and David E. Rogers fault the media for contributing to the initial delay. They report that the media initially ignored the epidemic. The media, they point out, "frame issues for the public and often help determine the political agenda for our nation. Government responses frequently depend on attitudes generated by media attention, and numerous studies have shown that people get many of their facts, ideas, and attitudes toward social issues from television, newspapers, and magazines. In this instance, the press and the media did little to encourage a swift public response" (1990:110).[11]

The hesitant response to AIDS was not limited to the United States. The initial reaction in Sweden and the United Kingdom was also "slow and cautious, even dilatory in the eyes of some" (Fox et al.

---

[11] Using a historical perspective, both Swenson (1988) and Rosenberg (1990) note that denial, slow acceptance, and delay in the official response to epidemic have been common occurrences. Cholera in nineteenth century New York City and influenza in France, Spain, and the United Kingdom in 1918 are cited as examples.

1990:310), as it was also in France and Italy, where most AIDS cases had first occurred among drug addicts.[12]

The reasons for the delayed response in the United States are complex and varied. According to the first report of the Institute of Medicine (1986b),[13] an analytic appraisal of the first years of the epidemic, initial efforts to develop consistent public health policies were hampered by lack of knowledge of the nature of the new disease. The lack of information nurtured what proved to be an unwarranted optimism that once the biomedical scientists had identified the cause of the disease, treatment and vaccines would soon follow.

Osborn (1990), on the other hand, blames the underestimation of the menace of AIDS on the scientific community's unbridled optimism that science and technology would solve the problem. Episodes of epidemic infectious diseases such as legionnaires' disease and toxic shock syndrome had been dealt with successfully, and it was tempting to assume that it was only a matter of time before AIDS would also be conquered. Moreover, as Fox (1988a) pointed out, by the 1980s dealing with infectious disease had become a routine process that absorbed less than 5 percent of public health funds. In fact, the problem of epidemic infectious disease was seen as a concern only to the developing world.

A major factor determining the response of the American health polity,[14] according to Fox, was that it was influenced by the political priorities of the Reagan administration. The primary emphasis of the administration was on dealing with chronic degenerative illness because of the declining importance of infectious diseases. The dominant philosophy was to foster individual responsibility for health. Furthermore, the Reagan administration was reluctant to turn to Congress for funds to support AIDS research and services because of the root causes of the disease as it manifested itself in the United States, that is, in dangerous sex practices and in infection through drug injections. Moreover, Fox maintains that the institutions and the leaders at the forefront of

---

[12] Rosenberg (1990:4) remarks dryly that "bodies must accumulate and the sick must suffer in increasing numbers before officials acknowledge what can no longer be ignored."

[13] Based on presentations at the annual meetings of the Institute of Medicine in October 1985 in Washington, D.C.

[14] Fox uses the term *health polity* to designate the individuals, policies, and institutions that conceive and organize responses to health and illness.

health affairs were "poorly prepared to take aggressive, confident action against an infectious disease that was linked in the majority of cases to individual behavior, was expensive to study and treat, and required a coordinated array of public and personal health services" (1988a:316).

A second report of the Institute of Medicine (1986a), by a committee headed by the Nobel laureate David Baltimore, made a more alarming appraisal of the emerging seriousness of the epidemic and outlined a range of public health measures that it deemed essential to control it. Noting the mounting pressure on the health care system, it stressed contingency long-range planning and it called for a massive educational campaign to prevent infection that would stress the need for using latex condoms in sexual relations to prevent infection. It did not, however, deal with what has since emerged as a crucial question in reaching the public through mass education programs—namely, how effective such messages would be in altering the risky behavior that causes HIV infection.

The most telling criticisms of the AIDS effort, however, have come from the two presidential advisory commissions on the HIV epidemic. The first, headed by Admiral James R. Watkins, is the Presidential Commission on the Human Immunodeficiency Virus Epidemic, which issued a report (1988) describing the epidemic as being more serious than had been initially perceived and stressing its changing nature, that is, its growing concentration among disadvantaged groups such as black and Hispanic minorities, the homeless, and poor women, as well as among homosexuals. It criticized the management of the epidemic under the Reagan administration. Its specific targets of criticism were (1) the search for drugs to treat the disease and for a vaccine to prevent it by the Federal Drug Administration—which it criticized as being slow and disorganized, and (2) the entire public health effort for lack of uniform and strong antidiscrimination laws that were needed to protect the victims of AIDS.

The second commission, appointed in August 1989 by President Bush, with public health physician June E. Osborn as chair, was the National Commission on Acquired Immune Deficiency Syndrome. This commission was given the mandate of "promoting the development of a national consensus" on policy concerning AIDS. In two interim reports, the commission was even more critical of the government's record in coming to grips with the full dimensions of the AIDS problem. Its first report (1989: 2) sounded these warnings:

- There is a "dangerous, perhaps growing complacency toward an epidemic that many people want to
  believe is over."
- The epidemic is reaching "crisis proportions among
  the young, the poor, women, and many minority
  communities" and the situation will grow much
  worse in the 1990s.
- The link between drug use and HIV infection "must
  be acknowledged and addressed in any national
  drug strategy."
- "There is no national plan for helping the faltering
  health care system to deal with the impact of the HIV
  epidemic."

The commission's second interim report (1990a:2) assailed
the lack of leadership that has characterized the AIDS effort,
comparing it to "an orchestra without a conductor," in which the
participants were all playing their own tune—"sometimes we har-
monize, sometimes we don't." While acknowledging the periodic and
creative efforts to address the HIV epidemic at every level of
government, it nonetheless described the need for coordinating
these efforts. Coordination, the commission believes, is the missing
link to an effective and cohesive national strategy and of a clear
cooperative plan that would make responsible use of the limited
funds available.

In other interim reports, the commission covered a range of
issues: AIDS and the workforce in rural America (August 1990b);
HIV in correctional institutions (March 1991); the relationship
between substance abuse and HIV infection (July 1991); HIV
transmission in health care settings (1992a); and AIDS among
minorities (1992b). In a major report (1991c), entitled *America Living
with AIDS: Transforming Anger, Fear, and Indifference into Action,*[15]
the commission indicted the government's response to the AIDS
crisis:

> Our nation's leaders have not done well. In the past
> decade, the White House has rarely broken its silence
> on the topic of AIDS. Congress has shown leadership in
> developing critical legislation, but has often failed to
> provide adequate funding for AIDS programs. Articu-

---

[15] The recommendations in the interim reports are included in the Appendix
of this report.

late leadership guiding Americans toward a greater response to AIDS has been notably absent. We are accustomed to hearing from the "bully pulpit" about national problems and how we should address them, so perhaps the public cannot be blamed for assuming that such a silence means that nothing important is happening. Their false calm is reinforced by politicians who claim that enough has been done about AIDS, since it is "just one disease," and that we should redirect our attention to other diseases that currently kill more people (National Commission on AIDS 1991c:3).

The commission's critique, widely reported in the national press, was made more dramatic by the public resignation from the commission of the basketball star player Earvin "Magic" Johnson, a year after his appointment to the Commission by President Bush— on the basis of Johnson's public announcement that he had tested HIV-positive. Johnson accused the Bush administration of having "utterly ignored" the commission's recommendations for further aggressive efforts to combat the epidemic.

Criticisms pointing to belated, disjointed, and inadequate efforts are the ones most often repeated by critics, as noted by Padraig O'Malley (1989). But the root causes of this state of affairs seem to be more complex than a mere failure of political will or intent, of misperception of the magnitude of the AIDS problem, or of willful neglect. The failures, according to other analysts, are based in defects of the system that deals with public health. One analysis of these systemic flaws provides insights into the decision-making processes. Sandra Panem, who was trained as a virologist, has analyzed the structure of government agencies on which American society relies in a health emergency (1988). Her central thesis is that lack of leadership in the AIDS effort is a function of a lack of clear-cut divisions of responsibility among federal, state, and local levels of authority. As a result, patient care strategies and the delivery of health services have lagged behind research and epidemiology. Compounding these difficulties is the lack of communication among the various layers and components of the health establishment and the fact that—especially at the beginning of the epidemic—the Public Health Service[16] was short of senior personnel and was

---

[16] The U.S. Public Health Service is a component of the Department of Health and Human Services; the Centers for Disease Control and Prevention (CDC) in Atlanta, Georgia, is an agency of the Public Health Service.

seriously underfunded. (It had only 3 percent of the budget allocated to the Department of Health and Human Services, although it was responsible for the major part of the problem of dealing with the AIDS crisis.)[17] In a foreword to Panem's book, Samuel O. Thier (1988:6), then president of the Institute of Medicine, defined the organizational dilemma that has caused the inadequate response to AIDS—"the most serious epidemic to face the country in decades"— as the sum of the independent responses of the many components of our health and social systems.[18]

Sociologists Perrow and Guillén (1990) analyzed the slow response to the AIDS crisis from the standpoint of organizational dynamics. Not only governmental but also private organizations were slow to react to the mounting threat. Basing their analysis on the response of New York City, one of the hardest hit urban centers in the United States, they indict the paucity of strong indigenous community groups and their failure, along with government agencies, to provide the necessary education and care in response to the AIDS epidemic.

The counter-critique by conservatives

Criticism has also come from conservatives who are generally unenthusiastic about government initiatives and have in this instance challenged the generally liberal assumptions that AIDS constitutes a major crisis and that the government has been indifferent or apathetic toward it.

A major figure in this conservative criticism has been Michael Fumento, who ridiculed the widely respected Harvard paleontologist and geologist Stephen Jay Gould (calling him a "pop scientist") for writing in 1987 that "Yes, AIDS may run through the entire population, and may carry off a quarter or more of us." Fumento claimed that "statistics are doctored, homosexual demographics are overstated, and scarce research funds are squandered—all for an epidemic that may have peaked some time ago" (1989:21).

In his 1990 book, *The Myth of Heterosexual AIDS*, Fumento developed his argument further, asserting that the AIDS epidemic had become a national priority far out of proportion to its actual

---

[17] For an overview of the organization of U.S. government agencies involved in public health activities, see Chapter 2 in Panem (1988).

[18] For a detailed analysis of the recent history of U.S. health policy and its relevance to AIDS, see Fox (1988a).

danger to the population at large—particularly to white, hetero-sexual, middle class, mainstream Americans. Calling for an end to the AIDS hysteria which he claims has siphoned off research funds, he maintained that people will die of other diseases that have had less success than AIDS has had in obtaining federal funding for research (Fumento 1990).

Although Fumento has been the most visible of the conserva-tive critics, he is not alone. A number are cited by Timothy F. Murphy (1991) in a review article entitled "No Time for an AIDS Backlash." Murphy, a medical educator at the University of Illinois College of Medicine, criticizes Charles Krauthammer, who had written in *Time* magazine that "AIDS has become the most privileged disease in America." Similarly, Murphy criticized the *Chicago Tribune* colum-nist Mike Royko for his views that the sums spent on AIDS research are excessive and that some AIDS education posters have far more to do with the promotion of homosexuality than with the prevention of disease.

Reviewing the critique of the response to AIDS can obscure the remarkable positive initial accomplishments of the public health effort: (1) the record-breaking rapid identification of the human immunodeficiency virus as the causative agent of the disease by scientists at the National Institutes of Health and the Pasteur Institute in Paris; (2) the analytic epidemiological studies that documented the mode of transmission and the prevalence of infection both in the United States and in other countries; (3) the development by the Centers for Disease Control of an effective system of surveil-lance of AIDS cases (Kuller & Kingsley 1986); and (4) the develop-ment of serological tests to monitor the epidemic and to protect the supply of donated blood (Osborn 1990).[19] These are all evidence of the successful application by scientists and public health experts of traditional public health approaches to epidemic control.

Cross-national analyses of responses to AIDS

A growing body of literature seeks to examine and evaluate the response of countries throughout the world to the epidemic. The following are representative examples of these analyses.

Two collections of essays—*Action on AIDS: National Policies in Comparative Perspective*, edited by two scholars at Griffiths Univer-sity in Brisbane, Australia, Barbara A. Misztal and David Moss

---

[19] The testing of blood donors is now mandated in the United States and in most other industrialized countries.

(1990), and *AIDS in the Industrialized Democracies: Passions, Politics, and Policy*, edited by David L. Kirp, at the Graduate School of Public Policy, University of California, Berkeley, and Ronald Bayer of the Columbia School of Public Health (1992)—provide analyses of the worldwide response to the epidemic. *Action on Aids* contains essays on Africa, Australia, Belgium, Brazil, France, Italy, Poland, the United States, and West Germany; and *AIDS in the Industrialized Democracies* includes essays on Australia, Canada, Denmark, France, Germany, Japan, the Netherlands, Spain, Sweden, the United Kingdom, and the United States.

Action on AIDS emphasizes contrasts in the social and epidemiological profiles of countries in both the developed and the developing world that governed their response to AIDS; *AIDS in the Industrialized Democracies* focuses exclusively on AIDS policy and politics in the economically advanced countries.

In the concluding chapter of their book (Chapter 11, 235–249), Misztal and Moss present what they call "an interim report" on how AIDS was managed in the first decade of its appearance. From their analysis of the responses to AIDS in eight countries and the sub-Saharan African region, they reach a number of conclusions. Among them are the following:

- The formulation of national strategies to deal with AIDS has been cautious.
- In some instances, inaction has been judged to be justified in dealing with a health problem initially associated with marginalized and stigmatized groups.
- Some governments have backed away from instituting measures known to be unenforceable.
- The symbolic power of national political initiatives has been invoked sparingly in dealing with the "taboo" issues involved in AIDS.

The editors isolate seven key factors that must be considered as having influenced AIDS policies:

1. *The primacy of international relations.* National AIDS policies are influenced by foreign relations. France was motivated by national pride to display a humane response. Poland's response was influenced by its desire to match the civility of other nations. The rhetoric of Australia's health officials often referred to Australia's leadership role. The first meeting of the two Germanies after unification led to an agree-

ment to collaborate in AIDS research.

2.   *The changing social profile of AIDS.* In each country, HIV infection has been linked to particular social groups: homosexuals in the United States, intravenous drug users in Italy, prostitutes in Central Africa, foreign students in Belgium and Eastern Europe. Changes in the vulnerability of these groups—some gradual, as in the United States, and some more rapid, as in Brazil and France, where AIDS is spreading among the lower middle and lower classes— create problems requiring governmental response.

3.   *The social identity of groups at risk.* Singling out high-risk groups intensifies stigmatization. In Brazil, the identity of subgroups at risk of AIDS is made difficult by the ambiguity of the term *partner*, which blurs sexual identity among homosexuals and bisexuals.

4.   *The extent of organization in high-risk communities.* Gay organizations in France and the United States have had a significant impact on AIDS policies. In Poland, in sharp contrast, governmental harassment and church-inspired disapproval have prevented gays from becoming organized.

5.   *The participatory traditions of civil society.* Voluntary associations are key components of American society; self-help groups and collective efforts in the area of health are traditional and have provided networks of support in the AIDS epidemic. At the other end of the continuum are postcolonial African societies, where civil wars and communal violence have been destructive of collective efforts. European countries occupy different positions between these two extremes. In Poland, for example, collective initiatives can only take place in the "interstices" or if "camouflaged within" existing state institutions. Volunteer efforts and pressure to influence governmental action exist—but only within the state's central role in protecting social welfare.Voluntary associations are weak in Italy but much stronger in Germany, the Netherlands, and Switzerland.

6. *The extent of political consensus.* A consistent theme of the response to AIDS in these countries is that AIDS has not entered into domestic politics. Few of the contentious issues involved divide along party or ministerial lines; committees formed to deal with AIDS have been bipartisan or nonpolitical. This has been true of countries with a narrow political spectrum—such as Belgium, the United States, and West Germany—as well as of those countries with a wide political spectrum with extremes from left to right, such as France and Italy. Political consensus has predominated in most instances in most countries.

7. *The resources and structure of the medical system.* Both HIV and AIDS are the responsibility of a country's medical services. Many countries classify them both as sexually transmitted diseases, but treatment centers for STDs are chronically underfunded and the burden of care thus falls on hospitals. Governments have responded to pressure and have increased funding for both hospitals and specialized treatment centers. The decentralized character of the medical system in the United States provides both flexibility and local autonomy in the delivery of health care, but it is not economical and health services vary widely in scope and quality. Furthermore, the system requires supplemental services by both volunteers and the afflicted. The growing refusal of private insurers to enroll HIV-infected persons generates higher hospital costs.

Kirp and Bayer (1992) present a different rationale for their cross-national comparative analysis. They restrict themselves to examining AIDS policy and politics in eleven economically advanced and democratic nations. Their purpose is to determine how different national cultures have affected the response to AIDS and have shaped the experience of the epidemic, even when embedded in economic systems that are able to provide decent (if not always equitable) health care. They examine the following topics in the development of AIDS policy:

- Public health traditions concerning mandatory

measures (testing, screening, reporting of disease carriers, contact tracing) and the history of efforts on the part of public health officials to retain the full exercise of public health powers.

- The nature and management of measures to control drug use; their status in criminal law; and the nature of treatment programs.
- The legal status of homosexuality and protections against discrimination; the degree of organization in the gay community; and the forms of opposition to homosexuality.
- The status of sex education in public schools and other institutions and the extent to which moralistic concerns have influenced this education.
- The status of the confidentiality of medical reports; whether or not they are protected by custom or law; and the status of national policies on discrimination and the identity of the groups protected.
- Health and social security; the question of who bears the cost of illness in the society; whether the system of health insurance extends to long-term home care; and whether there is continuum of care givers for dealing with chronic disease.
- The policymaking process; the presence or absence of a tradition of consultation or formal cooperation with interest group constituencies in the formulation and implementation of health and social policy.

The authors caution that policy decisions on AIDS in any country cannot be characterized by single, simple formulations. Nonetheless, it is possible to identify two policy approaches. One, a *contain-and-control* approach, stresses the compulsory identification and isolation of the HIV-infected. The other, a *cooperation-and-inclusion* approach, stresses cooperation with those who are most vulnerable to AIDS through education and voluntary testing and counseling—combined with guarantees of privacy.

Each of the industrialized democracies, the authors maintain, has had to make decisions concerning which elements of these contrasting policies it would adopt. The decisions made reflect the balance of political forces in the nation, the dominant values concerning privacy, the degree of commitment to personal liberty, and the value placed upon volunteerism—all in the context of the changing profile of AIDS. "In short," they conclude, "the politics of

AIDS is the politics of democracy in the face of a critical challenge to communal well being" (Kirp & Bayer 1992:5).

The international influence of U.S. AIDS policy

In a concluding chapter, Kirp and Bayer (1992:361–384) provide the following perspectives on the U.S. response to the AIDS crisis.

1. The United States, the nation with the largest concentration of cases in the Western world, became a pioneering model for confronting AIDS. As epidemiological patterns that were first observed in the United States manifested themselves in other countries, the American experience was seen as embodying the hopes of the other democracies for humane treatment and a quick cure. During the first decade of the epidemic, the authors state, "the United States produced the very best policy—and the very worst" (361).

2. The U.S. epidemiological model for tracing the diffusion of AIDS was adopted throughout the world.

3. Many elements of the AIDS policy adopted by the industrialized democracies by the end of the decade originated in the United States: blood screening, HIV testing and screening, and community-based prevention programs. The European countries adopted the system of voluntary groups providing medical care to the sick partly subsidized by the government.

4. Care-givers and pressure groups in Australia, Canada, Denmark, France, Germany, the Netherlands, and the United Kingdom adopted the American "buddy" system for the care of ailing victims—a system pioneered by the Gay Men's Health Crisis. The confrontational tactics used by American activists to protest what they called official inaction on AIDS and to accuse pharmaceutical companies of profiteering, the authors report, have been adopted worldwide.

5. On the research frontier, European scientists used many leads from American AIDS research (362); Australians participated in American-developed proposals; and other countries waited for American

research findings such as the one resulting in the adoption of the drug AZT for HIV-infected individuals. Findings from U.S. research journals were translated into a dozen or so languages.

Human rights policies in France, the United States, and the United Kingdom

Using a narrower range of analysis than that of the two books described above, an essay by the ethicist Carol A. Tauer (1988) focuses on the responses of France, the United Kingdom, and the United States to a number of bioethical issues involved in dealing with the problems of controlling the spread of AIDS. Although the United States and the countries of Western Europe subscribe to the same international declaration of human rights, Tauer notes, there are both conceptual and practical differences in their respective understanding of these statements. In considering the human rights aspects of AIDS, it is necessary to consider the influence of different legal concepts and cultural values. Issues such as privacy, confidentiality, informed consent, and the right to know entail different legal interpretations and different culturally based attitudes toward doctor–patient relations. The much discussed (but rarely invoked) use of quarantine—historically a classic public health strategy—involves an interpretation of human rights. And the problem of how to inform and educate the public also involves different culturally rooted value judgments.

In the United States there is general agreement on the issue of patients' rights, such as informed consent and the right to be informed of a medical diagnosis or prognosis. In France and the United Kingdom, however, there is a more paternalistic conception of physician–patient relations; for example, in court cases, French and British judges defer almost exclusively to the medical profession. Clinical issues in Britain, Tauer reports, remain under the jurisdiction of the Medical Council.

Voluntary testing and screening for HIV infection is recommended policy in the United States as an outgrowth of the "right-to-know" principle. In contrast, public health authorities in the United Kingdom did not urge antibody tests for HIV infection even for members of high-risk groups—in the interests of protecting the confidentiality of the data.

Tauer emphasizes that concepts concerning the protection of civil rights differ from country to country and that "these differences engender subtle variations in the national concern for the civil rights of AIDS victims" (165). France and the United Kingdom subscribe to the Convention on Human Rights of the European Community, which provides explicit protection to the privacy of individuals and families. Observers have noted, Tauer reports, that Europeans at risk of AIDS are relatively unconcerned about the possible loss of their civil rights. This may reflect the fact that homosexual behavior is generally not illegal in Europe. Furthermore, the national health care systems of most European countries provide health care to all their citizens.

Kirp and Bayer document another key element in the struggle against AIDS, one also noted by Misztal and Moss: the role of homosexual voluntary associations. The activities of the Gay Men's Health Crisis in the United States (in the cities of New York and San Francisco) have been widely emulated in Australia, Canada, Denmark, France, Germany, the Netherlands, and the United Kingdom. In France, "the transformation of the AIDS problem from a particular issue into a general cause" Pollak (1990:85) says, "can be described sociologically as a process of alliance building between the gay associations and the world of the health professionals." The associations served as conduits to the groups most at risk and most difficult to reach. Subsequently, these groups became part of a worldwide movement to protest both the inaction of officials and the actions of pharmaceutical firms that were accused of profiteering on death. The motto "Silence = Death" became an international slogan of gay associations (Kirp & Bayer 1992:362).

The key role played by self-help groups in many European countries is even more developed in Australia, according to Dennis Altman (1991:10). In some ways, Altman says, "the threefold partnership achieved between the government, community groups, and health professionals is a model for many similar countries." The Australian government has funded a national organization—the Australian Federation of AIDS Organizations—which provides representation for the entire range of affected communities.

One outstanding conclusion that emerges from these cross-cultural comparisons of the responses of democratic societies to AIDS concerns the limits of political and social conservatism. Although the appearance of AIDS coincided with a period of political conservatism (e.g., Ronald Reagan in the United States and Margaret Thatcher in the United Kingdom) and of public expressions of homophobia, none of the industrialized democracies adopted or apparently even considered a truly coercive strategy against AIDS. However, the democratic nations differ considerably in their willingness to consider legislative provisions to control the spread of

AIDS. Australia, the United Kingdom, and the United States have all developed strategies to encourage behavioral change among the infected—stressing counseling-and-warning strategies, with restrictions placed on movement only as a last resort. Sweden has shown a greater willingness to consider restrictive measures. AIDS is included under the provisions of Swedish venereal disease laws, requiring compulsory testing; reporting of the infected to authorities; warnings given to sexual partners; prohibition of risky conduct; and, in certain cases, confinement to hospital (Tauer 1988). Patients are requested to sign a contract consenting to regular medical examinations, committing themselves to inform prospective sexual partners of their being infected, and informing all physicians and dentists of their condition (Earickson 1990).

The responses of countries around the world to AIDS reveal a basic dilemma: how to control the spread of the infection through the identification of risk groups and the actual carriers of the disease while at the same time preserving fundamental human rights to privacy, confidentiality, and freedom of movement. In the industrial democracies, a balance seems to have been found, and quarantine in the classic sense of isolation and restriction of movement has been rejected.

AIDS control in a dictatorship: The case of Cuba

Since all democratic nations have rejected the option of coercion as a means of controlling the spread of AIDS (Kirp & Bayer 1992:361–370), the case of Cuba provides a dramatic illustration of the response of a self-proclaimed nondemocratic society. Based on several descriptions and evaluations of the Cuban government's responses to the threat of AIDS (Bazell 1992; Earickson 1990; Mazur 1992; Misztal & Moss 1990; Pérez-Stable 1991), the following features of the Cuban response emerge.

Unlike other Caribbean countries, Cuba had experienced relatively few cases of AIDS; as of 1992, "only 773 HIV infections, 108 cases of full-blown AIDS, and 60 deaths" had been reported (Bazell 1992:14). One source of infection has been Cuba's recent military and political involvement in Africa; that is, AIDS has been imported by diplomats, soldiers, and students who participated in Castro's military and political adventures in Angola, Ethiopia, and Mozambique. Another source has been sexual relations b[e]Cuban women and bisexual men, who were themselves infe[cted]gay partners. Heterosexual anal intercourse is reported to hav[e]responsible for over half of the infections among women

Ministry of Public Health, MINSAP, denies the existence of any illicit intravenous drug use in Cuba; see Pérez-Stable 1991:563).

According to Pérez-Stable, a Cuban-American physician, MINSAP contends that mandatory lifetime quarantine is the only method of guaranteeing that HIV-infected persons will behave in a sexually responsible way. Its greatest fear is of irresponsible sexual behavior among men characterized by *machismo*—that is, men who are likely to seek extramarital sexual partners. He quotes a ministry spokesman who maintains that lifetime quarantine will "radically alter the threat of the HIV epidemic in Cuba by restricting the personal liberty of these individuals" (564).

Cuba's strategy for controlling the spread of AIDS has been to test the entire adult population and to restrict all persons found to be seropositive to special residential parks located in rural areas. The parks are said to have better than average nutritional levels, medical care, and recreational facilities. Park residents receive their full salaries; the unemployed are given a stipend. Quarantine is obligatory, but the policy of isolation has been liberalized over the years. Patients with families close by are permitted weekend passes. Others may go home once a month. Patients exhibiting responsible behavior go to their regular jobs. They can be visited by relatives and friends and they can go on excursions to places of historical, cultural, or social interest. Treatment and meals are free. According to Mazur, sanitarian policies have changed often in response to patients' requests and more family visits have been allowed, as has employment outside the sanitarium.

Evaluating Cuba's HIV policy, Pérez-Stable lists some of its positive attributes. First is the fact that the health authorities will have obtained a full epidemiological profile of the entire adult population. Health authorities generally recognize that Cuba has established a reliable system for gathering data—in sharp contrast to the incomplete and unreliable epidemiological data from other developing countries. Second, widespread testing has minimized infections by contaminated blood products. Third, prenatal screening makes it possible for infected women to have therapeutic abortions. Fourth, after mandatory testing, education efforts have been undertaken. Fifth, contact tracing has been carried out.

In assessing the Cuban policy, the Pan American Health Organization's representative, Fernando Zacarias, praised the superb medical and psychological support given to the HIV-infected and to AIDS patients, but stated that "there is still a need to take a hard look at the human rights issue" (quoted in Mazur 1992: 9). Pérez-Sable maintains that, although compulsory testing may seem justifiable for public health reasons, little else can be said in defense of lifelong quarantine: there is little basis to justify this drastic measure, he believes (1991:564–565). And aside from its ethical drawbacks, the policy has fostered the idea among Cubans that MINSAP is responsible for taking care of their health and thus "removes the responsibility of behavioral change from the individual." Moreover, the policy may "paradoxically permit most Cubans to feel that they are personally invulnerable to the HIV epidemic" (1991:564565). In fact, according to Mazur, Cubans seem to accept the policy, having become used to the idea that the state is responsible for maintaining the health of the public.

7

The Task of Changing Social Behavior

Prospects for Stemming the Pandemic

The second decade of the pandemic has brought quantum leaps in the accumulation of biological knowledge about the dynamics of HIV infection and AIDS illness. Nonetheless, it is becoming increasingly apparent that, despite this progress, the prospects are bleak both for neutralizing the effects of HIV infection in individuals and for slowing the spread of the pandemic before the end of the century by biological intervention. This is the conclusion of the articles in a special issue of *Science* ("AIDS: The Unanswered Questions," May 28, 1993) which summarize the nature of the uncertainties faced by the international AIDS research community in its quest both for preventive vaccines and for clinical therapies that delay the onset and attenuate the severity of symptoms.

Uncertainty was the keynote of a survey of 150 leading AIDS researchers throughout the world undertaken by *Science* to assess the current status of the search for a cure for AIDS or for a vaccine to prevent it. The message *Science* received was "the more we learn, the less certain we are" (*Science*, AIDS Research, May 28, 1993:1254-1257).

Reviewing current knowledge concerning the treatment of HIV infection and the prospect for therapies, Marjorie I. Johnston and David F. Hoth (1993), scientists at the National Institute of Allergy and Infectious Diseases, arrived at the following conclusions: (1) despite advances in the development of experimental anti-HIV drugs, clinical therapy remains largely palliative, and (2) the emerging data on the pathology of immune reactions raises the possibility that even if the virus is eliminated from HIV-infected individuals, their immune systems will remain compromised.

Reporting on the search for a vaccine, Barton F. Haynes (1993) of the Duke Center for AIDS Research warned that "as yet there is no preventive vaccine on the near horizon with clear prospects for clinical use" (1279). The pace of the epidemic has forced the simultaneous investigation of several vaccine tracks: in 1993, there were some 16 candidate vaccines being tested in clinical trials in the United States, Europe, and Africa (1282). The term "vaccine," Haynes points out, is synonymous in the public mind with the notion of safety from infection. But in the case of AIDS it is very likely that most HIV vaccines will be less than 100 percent efficacious. (Recent analysis has suggested that the earlier use of a vaccine that is only 60 percent effective would prevent more new infections than the later use of a more efficient vaccine.)

Aside from describing the scientific complexities of developing a successful preventive vaccine, Haynes emphasizes that there are also many complex social and ethical issues involved in conducting clinical trials of candidate vaccines and particularly in conducting such trials in developing countries (1282). One thorny problem associated with vaccine trials is that immunization with experimental HIV immunogens results in seropositivity to HIV testing among the participants. Protection of these uninfected vaccine trial participants from social discrimination, Haynes speculates, may become difficult. Another paradoxical outcome of the trials is the possibility that participation by volunteers—by creating among them a false sense of security—could result in an increase in their high-risk behavior.

The magnitude of the social problems of testing a preventive vaccine on an international scale is the concern of Michael H. Merson (1993). No preventive vaccine, Merson insists, will have a significant impact unless it is appropriate for both developed and developing countries. Because 90 percent of all new infections by the year 2000 will occur in the developing world, an initial mass immunization campaign in the high-prevalence countries will need to reach over 300 million people during the first five years alone. Low-cost vaccines will be needed in the developing world, where there will also be problems of transport and storage.

A complicating factor in future vaccine use will be the need to protect people from a variety of HIV strains. Above all, says Merson, a vaccine will have to induce long-lasting immunity with few doses. Vaccine field trials will have to respect community traditions. (Four trial sites have already been selected in Brazil, Rwanda, Thailand, and Uganda.) Merson also warns, furthermore, that no preventive vaccine is likely to be 100 percent effective. Total population coverage is difficult to achieve, as has been shown during decades of experience with vaccines against childhood diseases.

For all these reasons, it is now widely recognized by biological as well as social scientists that a preventive vaccine—the ultimate "tech-fix" solution—can complement but cannot replace other methods of prevention. "The prevention agenda for the 1990s and beyond," Merson emphasizes, "thus calls for continued reliance on our ability to convince and enable people to avoid risky sexual behavior and to ensure that they are treated promptly and effectively for conventional STDs" (1267).

In reviewing the achievements of research on AIDS, Oliver Morton and his colleagues (1992:231) observe that while science seeks a cure or a vaccine, "prevention and behavioral research must bear a large share of the responsibility for slowing the spread of AIDS."

Prevention, however, has not been a top priority throughout the world. As Lars O. Kallings pointed out at the 1993 Berlin meetings, "the AIDS epidemic is an emergency, but society is responding as if it were not" (New York Times, June 15, 1993:C1). Yet health workers in the field have emphasized the multiplier effect of prevention: each case prevented reduces the chances of additional cases and more deaths. James W. Curran, who directs the AIDS program at the CDC, urged the convening of a national meeting in the United States devoted solely to prevention, bringing together disparate groups devoted to family planning, the treatment of STDs, and HIV prevention (New York Times, June 15, 1993:C1).

The prevention effort is composed of many approaches and objectives. These range from direct, face-to-face interventions—by social workers and medical personnel—with intravenous drug users and persons infected with STDs, to broad-scale education campaigns directed at the public at large. The paradox of HIV infection is that on the surface it is the most easily avoidable of all lethal infections, since acquiring it is the result of known, specific forms of behavior. Furthermore, the use of a simple barrier device during intercourse, that is, the condom, is known to be quite effective, as is the use of a sterile needle during an intravenous drug injection. Thus, changing the patterns of risky behavior that prevail among members of specific groups (homosexuals, bisexuals, intra-venous drug users, and adolescents) and preventing vulnerable behavior in the heterosexual population at large are the avowed goals of public education programs. But although there is broad consensus about the goals of educational programs designed to control the epidemics in both the developed and the developing world, dissension and controversy swirl around the specific objectives, appropriate targets, and nature of the messages to use. According to Jonathan Mann and his colleagues (1992), the world's efforts to induce behavioral change are handicapped by disagreements concerning sex education, condom distribution, and needle exchange programs. In their book, they deplore the enormous discrepancies between the industrialized and the developing countries in the funding for AIDS prevention programs. They note that only 6 percent of worldwide expenditures for AIDS prevention are spent in the developing world—which accounts for 80 percent of all HIV infections (321).

The formidable task of preventing AIDS through education throughout the world encounters two categories of obstacles. Some are rooted in society—in ideology, in politics, in religion, in moral and cultural values. But others—perhaps the most intractable—are rooted in individual psychology, in the most intimate recesses of behavior: sexual preferences, urges, and impulses.

The Societal Context of AIDS Education

AIDS education in the United States

The initial targets of AIDS education in the United States—male homosexuals—constituted an essentially cohesive and middle-class subculture skilled at collective action to obtain political objectives: many had had experience in creating the so-called gay liberation agenda (Altman 1988). Accordingly, information campaigns to change risky sexual practices, undertaken by voluntary associations of gays in collaboration with public health authorities, have so far been assessed as successful in stemming the tide of new cases.[1] As a result, HIV transmission among older men has been sharply reduced from the early 1980s; however, it continues at high levels among younger gay men. As the final report of the National

---

[1] Gay organizations like the Gay Men's Health Crisis have set up services and support structures that are models for other groups facing similar catastrophes in the future, according to Poirier (1988).

Commission on AIDS (1993:6) observes, a "generation gap" seems to have led to the rejection of warnings from survivors of the first "tragic decade." And other vulnerable subgroups—principally minority homosexuals, bisexuals, and drug addicts (many of whom are homeless) and their heterosexual partners—present daunting problems.

According to Osborn (1990), the growing recognition that bisexuals may be playing a role in the spread of infection among heterosexuals is cause for worry, although very little is known about bisexuality, which she believes is a universal feature of human culture. Difficult to quantify, bisexual behavior constitutes a critical area of concern with serious implications for black and Hispanic communities.

The broader objective of preventing the type of behavior that can result in exposure to the virus among the population at large—heterosexuals, young adults, adolescents, children of school age, potential blood donors, and members of minority communities—requires a different dynamic and runs into a different category of problems. The Watkins report (Presidential Commission 1988) distinguished among three types of education: distinct subpopulation targeting, information aimed at the general population, and school-based education. It underscored a basic quandary in all three activities: how to provide explicit messages without appearing to promote risky behavior. It also affirmed that it is not the role of the federal government to dictate values to local communities. As with other aspects of the official response to the epidemic, the federal response to the need to mount educational campaigns is frequently criticized as having been delayed, hesitant, and haphazard. The 1989 report of the National Commission was even more critical of the government's educational efforts, saying that even the language of prevention is constrained in the name of morality.

In the United States, the laboratory research response to AIDS seems to have been better funded and more focused than parallel efforts in the sphere of education to change behavior and encourage prevention. For example, only 13 percent of the $1.08 billion 1993 AIDS budget of the National Institutes of Health was earmarked for prevention (Science, News & Comment, April 30, 1993:615). The prospect for a major government education effort has been controversial from the outset (Bayer 1989). As Kenneth Keniston (1990:xxxiii) observes dryly, "to call for safer nonmarital sex or safer IV drug use invites bitter political controversy, whereas to call for 'more biomedical research' is politically advantageous." In an editorial in the American Journal of Public Health, David E.

Rogers, vice chair of the National Commission on AIDS, offered a blistering critique of the Reagan–Bush era AIDS programs:

> We have failed to develop any national prevention program worthy of the name . . . We have allowed arguments about taste or morality or propriety to block the delivery of potentially lifesaving information and devices to our teenagers, to drug users, and to the American community at large . . . For sexually active youngsters, we have failed to supply explicit, unequivocal information about human reproduction, the value of stable relationships, and the use of condoms . . . For drug users, we have failed to develop clean-needle exchange programs . . . This administration has even put a roadblock in the way of behavioral studies that might tell us what our children are actually up to in their sexual lives—information that might help us design more effective prevention programs (1992:523).

Ideological opposition to educational programs

Despite widespread anxiety about the epidemic in the United States, once its full potential was realized and the need for information on how to avoid infection was generally accepted, outspoken and subtle opposition began to be offered to the explicit messages that the public health community deemed necessary to prevent risky behavior. The opposition has had a political, attitudinal, religious, and cultural base.

The opposition from political conservatives in the United States was headed by Senator Jesse Helms who proposed an amendment threatening to withhold funds for safer sex education programs sponsored by organizations receiving federal support. Subsequently modified, the AIDS bill was passed in 1988. Osborn (1990) notes that, although other federal agencies (such as the Department of Defense for military recruiting) use television spots, it is technically illegal for the U.S. Public Health Service to purchase prime time on television; therefore, public service announcements about AIDS are relegated to off-peak hours. The advocacy, by then Surgeon General C. Everett Koop, of explicit and early school-based education programs to combat the spread of AIDS was opposed by Secretary of Education William J. Bennett during the Reagan administration. According to Panem (1988), it was only in the sixth year of the epidemic that a significant congressional appropriation for AIDS education was allocated.

In marked contrast, Australia, Canada, the United Kingdom, and many other countries in Western Europe mounted sustained public education programs. Despite traditional British reticence, the U.K. government launched a national media campaign to change sexual behavior through explicit messages to reduce sexual promiscuity and to promote the use of condoms. Denmark, Germany, Italy, and Norway undertook equally aggressive and explicit campaigns (Aiken 1987; Osborn 1990).

The basic problem underlying the effort to contain the epidemic through education is the near-universal public dislike of the explicit messages deemed necessary to be effective. In the United Kingdom, for example, the government health campaign met with public hostility because its language was considered offensive (Porter & Porter 1988). In the United States, Osborn (1990) points out, there has been a fundamental ambivalence about discussions of sexuality, as is evident in the general avoidance of frank discussions on the topic in the family, despite the fact, ironically, that the public media are saturated with sexual innuendo.[2] Generic, incomplete, and ambiguous messages fostered confusion and misunderstanding, the report stated, while what was needed were unambiguous messages in unvarnished language. AIDS has exacerbated the long standing controversy in American society concerning the proper content of sex education in the schools. There has been continuing hostility toward contraceptive advice for teenagers despite—paradoxically—an epidemic of teenage pregnancy, the prevalence of abortion as a means of birth control, and an epidemic increase in sexually transmitted diseases. School boards continue to wrestle with the issue of whether or not to distribute condoms to students.

Fineberg (1988a) also sees the disagreements concerning the appropriateness of the messages necessary to prevent AIDS as stemming from deep-seated fears and inhibitions in American society. The moralist view condemns both sexual relations outside marriage and the use of drugs; therefore, recommending condoms and offering to exchange sterile for used needles are seen as condoning immoral acts. The rationalist view is that these behaviors are a reality and should be modified to make them safer. In between these philosophical positions are various shadings of points of view:

---

[2] The National Commission on AIDS, in its report *America Living with AIDS* (1991c), criticized early educational messages couched in euphemisms such as "exchange of bodily fluids" instead of "intercourse" as the source of HIV infection.

tolerance of sexual relations outside of marriage, yet condemnation of homosexuality; opposition to drugs because of their dangers apart from AIDS, and hence opposition also to teaching addicts to clean their equipment (or use substitute needles), since this could be interpreted as sanctioning drug use. At least, says Osborn (1990), AIDS and other sexually transmitted diseases are acknowledged to be public health problems, while drug abuse and addiction have been treated as legal matters to be dealt with punitively.

The issue of the appropriate content of preventive AIDS education has been as divisive within the Roman Catholic church as it has been in society at large. In November 1987, elected representatives at the United States Catholic Conference, in a policy paper entitled *The Many Faces of AIDS: A Gospel Response* (1987:15, 18), sought to clarify the Catholic position on the topic of AIDS. Reaffirming Catholic moral teaching on human sexuality as a "gift from God . . . to be genitally expressed only in a monogamous, heterosexual relationship of lasting fidelity in marriage," they recognized, nonetheless, that "some people will not act as they can and should"—that is, they will not refrain from the type of sexual and drug abuse behavior that can transmit AIDS. "In such situations," the report declared, "educational efforts, if grounded in the broader moral vision outlined above could include accurate information about prophylactic devices or other practices proposed by some medical experts as potential means of preventing AIDS."

The document stressed that the church is not promoting the use of prophylactics "but merely providing information that is part of the factual picture." While rejecting educational advice on "safe sex" as "at best only partially effective," it criticized it for not taking into account "either the real values that are at stake or the fundamental good of the human person." However, the statement noted that accurate information about prophylactic devices might be included in educational programs that also stressed values and sexual abstinence outside of marriage. Educational programs about AIDS were also recommended for Catholic schools, although no mention was made of condoms.

The report provoked sharp debate within the ranks of the Catholic clergy. Denunciations from leading conservative bishops and cardinals (O'Connor of New York, Law of Boston) followed. In November 1989, at a conference on AIDS in Rome, the pope, who had previously refused to make a declaration of policy with specific reference to AIDS because of its links with promiscuity, homosexuality, and drug abuse (*New York Times*, January 29, 1988:A1, A6), finally addressed the matter. He reaffirmed Catholic doctrine on contraception and opposition to the use of condoms, declaring that it was illicit to seek AIDS prevention "based on recourse to means and remedies that violate the authentic sense of human sexuality" (*New York Times*, November 16, 1989:A10).[3]

For Jonathan Mann, the stance of the Catholic church reinforces those social conditions in poor countries that are the major contributing factors to the rising death rate from AIDS among women. Women often have "little bargaining power" to negotiate the practice of safe sex with their partners. The pope, he maintains, "sides with uncooperative men. Rome bars condoms because they prevent conception: their use is sinful even when a partner is HIV-infected." "Isn't it time," Mann asks, "the Vatican opens its eyes to the reality of people's lives and to the life-shattering pandemic of AIDS? Far more important than a device for birth control, the condom in today's world is essential for death control. Sacrificing millions of lives to HIV infection by prohibiting the only effective preventive against sexual transmission is totally irresponsible." So, he continues, is opposition to sex education in schools. "Adolescents deprived of counseling in human sexuality are being condemned to a game of infection roulette" (*International Herald Tribune*, December 1–2, 1990).

The 1991 report of the National Commission on AIDS took an equally strong position, stating that

> AIDS education and prevention efforts continue to be stymied by an unwillingness to talk frankly about sexual and drug use behavior that risk the spread of HIV. Constraints on discussions of sex, whether imposed by law, political considerations, issues of morality, language, or culture, have been a substantial barrier to the creation and implementation of effective HIV prevention programs. There is a cruel irony at work here, for reticence about discussing sex has become an obstacle to the implementation of lifesaving prevention programs (National Commission on AIDS 1991c:21).

---

[3] For a more detailed articulation of the conservative Catholic stance on the controversy, see Hale (1988). For a detailed discussion of the impact of AIDS on the Catholic church; on the church's role in education, particularly in the Chicano community in Los Angeles; on church policy on HIV testing; and on the tension between Vatican doctrine and the work of local parishes among poor, ethnic minorities, see Chapter V in Berk (1988).

The report went on to say that governmental restrictions on the use of education and prevention funds were seriously impeding HIV control, were needlessly prolonging the AIDS epidemic, and should be removed immediately.

The task of education to prevent AIDS is not clear-cut. Commenting upon the 1993 appointment by President Clinton of an AIDS "czar" (Kristine M. Gebbie), Christopher H. Foreman, Jr. of the Brookings Institution pointed out the complexity of her task. Much of the public health research community is convinced that, given sufficient effort, AIDS can be conquered if it is viewed as a health issue, not a moral one. Foreman points out that "AIDS has never been just about disease control . . . Like birth control, abortion and the classic venereal diseases, it is also unavoidably bound up with sex and reveals our lack of a moral consensus" (Foreman 1993:A19).

In an editorial in the *American Journal of Public Health*, Anke A. Ehrhardt (1992), director of the HIV Center for Clinical and Behavioral Studies at Columbia's College of Physicians and Surgeons, analyzes some of the failures of AIDS prevention education in the United States. One fundamental cause of these failures is the sociopolitical struggle between public health "realists" and social scientists on one side and the "moralizers" of the religious and radical right on the other. The goal of the public health realists is to change sexual practices that place people at risk, a goal that excludes judgments of sexual behavior of any type—homosexual, extramarital, premarital, or marital. Although equally committed to stemming the spread of AIDS, the moralizers oppose a neutral stance. They see disease prevention as secondary to upholding moral principles.

The struggle between moralizers and realists has crippled education and prevention in the United States. Moralizers have impeded efforts to provide realistic education in schools, insisting on messages promoting sexual abstinence and condemning any use of condoms. "They require no evidence and indeed there is none," Ehrhardt stresses, "that sexually active young people will abstain from sex if told to do so" (1460). He remarks that "revirginization" is not a practical undertaking and maintains that the struggle between realists and moralizers must end if the spread of HIV/AIDS morbidity and mortality is to be contained.

AIDS education in the developing world

Religious and political opposition to explicit education messages has not been confined to the West and the response of African societies to the AIDS epidemic has developed quite differently from that of the rest of the world. Fortin (1990) stresses that the very nature of the epidemic poses the kind of problem African societies are least capable of solving: the modification of intimate behavior. Prevention strategies also come into conflict with arbitrary political territories established during the colonial era—territories that include linguistically distinct and sometimes hostile groups. Efforts to strengthen the state through these arbitrary political units necessarily threaten tribal values, cohesion, and authority. Furthermore, state-run educational programs may undermine the leadership of tribal communities.

Fortin cites Kenya as an example of this paradox. AIDS prevention programs in Kenya are in English or Swahili rather than in native African languages, and thus they run counter to tribal identity and reinforce the power of the state. "The closer prevention programs move to more local ways of speaking about sexuality," Fortin maintains, "the closer these programs come into direct conflict with broader state objectives" (227).

In stressing the complexity of the problem of education throughout Africa, Fortin points out that the AIDS campaign in Uganda should ideally be conducted in twenty-two different languages. Dilemmas arise when the tasks for which the state is obviously better equipped to handle (i.e., those that require standardized operations compatible with Western technology) clash with the skills of private local groups and tribal leaders, who may be better equipped for the task of AIDS education. The paradoxical conclusion articulated by Fortin is that the nature of AIDS, its magnifying effect on other illnesses, and the strategies required for its prevention place the African state in an arena of action in which it is least competent. In Zambia, as Earickson (1990) reports, conflicts between the church and the government developed when the Ministry of Health issued a controversial educational booklet for use in secondary schools. Church leaders objected to passages describing how the use of condoms could reduce the risk of infection for individuals leading risky life-styles. A Zambian Pentecostal bishop criticized the message, which he maintained was telling schoolchildren that they could practice sex before marriage as long as it was considered safe. Eighty clergymen advocated removing the offending sections from the booklet.

In Tanzania, where HIV infection is increasing at an alarming rate, some organizations oppose the distribution of condoms because of their presumed association with illicit sex. Consequently, educational messages fail to mention condom use as a preventive measure for those individuals who reject abstinence as an option (Muhondwa 1991).

The Republic of South Africa was initially indifferent to AIDS because of the belief that the disease was limited to homosexuals—but it is indifferent no longer. The subservient position of women and the belief that condoms are part of a white plot to keep the black population in check, as well as the resistance of traditional healers, have been contributing factors to the increased incidence of AIDS in South Africa (*New York Times*, March 16, 1993:A1).

The government of Zimbabwe—where the tide of HIV infection began later than in Uganda and Zaire but is rising rapidly—at first denied the severity of the problem. Later, however, it developed one of the frankest and most widespread campaigns in Africa. President Robert C. Mugabe, a Roman Catholic, has been personally opposed to advocating condom use but has nevertheless permitted their distribution. A long-standing reticence about AIDS education has been overcome—first for 16-year olds and now for 11- to 12-year olds. A newly appointed health minister, Dr. Timothy Stamps, stepped up the educational campaign following a projection of AIDS cases that predicted, in the absence of behavior change, that by 2017 in a population that by then would number 18 million, the number of deaths would equal the number of births (*New York Times*, April 12, 1992:18).

In Uganda, Anglican bishops advise young people to marry early and remain faithful to their spouses—not only for the sake of Christian morality, but also to avoid contracting AIDS. A conference of church leaders on the topic of AIDS prevention went even further, advocating that sex education should begin as early as ten years of age (*World AIDS*, November 1991).

In Pakistan, which still has a low rate of infection but is facing the prospect of a massive spread of AIDS, designing a prevention program for a conservative Islamic society has been difficult because health educators have generally resisted making public statements concerning private behavior ("Pakistani Enigma: AIDS Education" 1992). However, increasing awareness of the specter of AIDS epidemics has forced official accommodations to traditional reticence. In India, the Indian Council of Medical Research sponsors a program utilizing elements of the nation's religious and cultural tradition to control the spread of AIDS, in the belief that Western-style television programs and printed booklets would have little effect on people whose lives are shaped more by religion than by science ("Focus: India" 1991).

Ethnic and cultural barriers

Another formidable bloc of obstacles interfering with effective HIV/AIDS education—both to prevent and to change risky behavior—is based in ethnic and cultural norms. Americans as culturally diverse as blacks, Hispanics, and Asians—the last two themselves representing various cultures—seem to have one characteristic in common. According to both social scientists and experts involved in directing outreach programs throughout the United States, there is among these minorities a taboo against the open discussion of sexual matters. Among blacks, women are thirteen times more likely to succumb to AIDS than whites, but "the idea of sexual candor, or of sexual agendas, has been kept in the closet" (Porter 1989:373).

Among Asians and Pacific islanders—a diverse group including Cambodians, Chinese, Filipinos, Koreans, and Vietnamese, as well as Hawaiians, Polynesians, and other islanders—sexuality is not considered an appropriate topic for discussion (Lee & Fong 1990). Moreover, for the Catholics and Confucians among them, such discussion is even considered immoral. The Tagalog language of the Philippines reportedly does not even have formal terms for penis, vagina, and intercourse, forcing community health workers to use street language, which many people find offensive, or English terms, which they do not understand. Among Hispanics, an all-inclusive category that includes Spanish-speaking peoples from Mexico and Central and South America as well as Brazilians and the people of the Caribbean, communication about sexuality occurs only in indirect and nonverbal ways (de la Vega 1990).

The subordinate status of women is a complicating factor throughout Latino communities. Porter (1989) notes that for Latinas, discussing sexuality would be perceived as unfeminine and perhaps immoral. Ernesto de la Vega, program director for AIDS in the Americas at the Panos Institute, warns that when local public health minority outreach workers distribute condoms to Latinas on their education rounds, they may not realize that they may have placed these women at risk of being battered. The Citizens Commission (1989) report, citing a study by the psychologists Mays and Cochran (1988), also points out that discussing sexual practices and encouraging condom use with traditional Hispanic women fails to reflect the reality of their lives, since cultural norms demand that women should enter into marriage with little knowledge about sex. De la Vega (1990:4) remarks that not only do Hispanic women not talk about sex, but also "they find it is even too embarrassing to acknowledge that they are actually there—fully conscious and present—during 'the act.' " In these cultures, women are caught in a dilemma; they are expected to be both seductive and virginal, in need of male protection but strong enough to bear many children. Men, on the other hand, are expected to be sexually experienced before marriage. They are also considered vulnerable to extramarital sexual temptation. The notion of contraception is for the most part unpopular.

Research conducted by Dooley Worth (1990) found that the prime target of education aimed at heterosexuals should be women—particularly poor blacks and Latinas, who represent 70 percent of all female AIDS cases. The effect of AIDS on minority women and their responses to AIDS education are poorly understood. "Culturally-determined values," she maintains, "influence how individual perceptions of AIDS are selected, how attitudes toward high risk behavior are formed, how habits that characterize high risk behavior are developed and how risk reduction information will be processed" (111).

Education programs that do not take into account the concept of *machismo* are bound to fail. Among Puerto Ricans in New York City, *machismo* is responsible for the refusal of men to use condoms because they are unmanly or unnatural. Condom use is also felt to be unromantic: since romance is culturally linked with virility and impregnation, their use denotes a lack of seriousness which is equated with marriage and pregnancy. *Marianismo*, the female counterpart of *machismo*, exalts chastity and influences how girls are raised—that is, to be subservient to all men: fathers, brothers, uncles, and husbands. Combined with economic powerlessness and exposure to dangerous environments, Worth maintains, these cultural mores support women's beliefs that they are unable to control what happens to them. This belief is compounded by a belief in *fatalismo*, which is linked to Catholicism. Thus, submissive sex-role behavior is constantly reinforced.[4]

Worth also stresses the high degree of cultural variation among American, Caribbean, and Haitian black women which

---

[4] According to Gil (1990), there are many disheartening instances of the failure of AIDS education. One of the most dramatic is Puerto Rico, which in 1990 had a higher incidence rate (48 per 100,000) than any of the fifty U.S. states, as well as a disproportionate number of pediatric and adolescent victims. All this is the case in spite of the fact that prevention measures were launched soon after the AIDS crisis was recognized.

needs to be explored if AIDS preventive education programs are to succeed. Black women in the United States, she points out, are often studied within the context of "social problems" and are seen as "culturally inadequate" and "disorganized." "Too often," she says, "the behavior of black women is filtered through cultural stereotypes." AIDS education advocating safer sex, Worth cautions, "may threaten behavior that black women link with survival" (124–125).

A second attitude shared by black, Hispanic, and Asian/ Pacific islander subcultures is the rejection of homosexuality. Dalton (1990), as noted earlier, attributes the black community's slow response to the AIDS threat to a reluctance to be associated with what is widely perceived as a gay disease. Indeed, he notes that gay black writers are more apt to excoriate racism within the white gay community than to target homophobia within the straight black community. Many black homosexual men feign involvement with black women as cover. Among Hispanics, according to de la Vega (1990), homosexuality is closeted. The strong prejudice it arouses because of the *machismo* tradition among Latino heterosexuals contributes to bisexuality; bisexual behavior, he warns, may prove to be "the entrance door for HIV into mainstream Latino communities in the United States and into Southern Latino societies, if public health educators, here and abroad, do not recognize it and take appropriate action immediately" (6). In Latino culture, a distinction must be made between sexual behavior and sexual identity. In some groups, self-proclaimed heterosexuals may be bisexual in private. Both homosexuality and bisexuality "show their faces only briefly," usually under the influence of drugs or alcohol. Consequently, education aimed at discussing sexual behavior in the context of AIDS runs into major difficulties.

Although homosexuality is ubiquitous throughout Asia and the Pacific islands, according to Lee and Fong (1990), it is suppressed; most homosexuals are "in the closet." Although many marry and have children, they continue to engage in homosexual relations. Because of their low visibility, these men are hard to reach through education efforts. AIDS is perceived as a disease of white homosexuals, and the prevailing sentiment is that if Asians and Pacific islanders keep to themselves, AIDS can be avoided. The authors blame this perception for the reluctance of these communities to see the epidemic as a problem.

According to the Centers for Disease Control, the incidence of AIDS among a fourth ethnically distinct group—Native Americans (American Indians, Alaskan Natives, and native Hawaiians)—has been low, although cases have been reported in every region of the country. However, Ronald M. Rowell (1990), a public health specialist who is executive director of the National Native American AIDS Prevention Center, points out that data from two seroprevalence studies show that American Indians and Alaskan natives have higher rates of infection than what would have been expected from the number of reported cases. In California, in fact, the seropositivity rate almost ties that of blacks. Indian community leaders have responded well to the need for AIDS education, fearful of what Rowell terms the potential of another "demographic collapse" of the American Indian sector of the population as a result of AIDS. With the epidemic's tendency to strike at individuals in their most fecund years, a tribe's whole future is at risk.

The signal importance of taking culture into account in planning educational campaigns is pointed out by John Rutayuga (1992b), a Tanzanian physician who has conducted medical and social research on AIDS for a number of years. He states that prevention education founders when indigenous traditions are ignored and educators are insensitive. In a letter to the editor of *AIDS & Society* (1992a), he reports that villagers have complained that prevention programs do not relate to them. Condoms are alien intrusions. "Education for HIV prevention," Rutayuga maintains, "is about nothing less than life and culture, and in Africa, references to these elements cannot be made except in the context of the family." The family has been underutilized, if not marginalized, by prevention programs in Africa, programs that have too often presented messages in a "colonial, pedagogical" manner. "Education for HIV prevention has to take people as they are and in their own environment" (2), Rutayuga concludes.

The Individual Context of AIDS Prevention

Life-style dynamics

Critics of AIDS prevention education maintain that, to be effective, messages must surmount life-style patterns that are intrinsic to subcultures in all societies. Rootless, often dictated by necessity rather than conviction, and often shifting, these life-styles are resistant to directed change. A report issued by UNICEF on "Street Youth and AIDS" (1993:1) presents a disheartening picture of the life-style of an increasing number (estimated to be in the millions) of children and youth living and working on the streets of large cities throughout the world—a life-style that makes them extremely vulnerable to AIDS. The increasing amount of research and publications describing this phenomenon provides only meager information about health. AIDS is seen as "a tremendous challenge" to workers with street youth in Brazil, Colombia, and Guatemala in particular. The report quotes from the words of youths themselves:

- When asked about AIDS, a 15-year-old Guatemalan responded: "Why should I care about AIDS? If I get infected today, I may die in seven years. So what? I could die tomorrow."
- A young Filipina stated: "AIDS might make me sick one day, but if I don't work my family would not eat and we will all be sick anyway."

The pandemic is seen as having a direct effect on young lives in many countries by creating a greater demand for young sex partners. As noted earlier, the market for sexual exploitation of children and youth is growing rapidly because clients believe that children are less likely to be infected with AIDS.

The resistance of the young to alter their life-style is universal, as illustrated by an anecdote reported by Earickson (1990:957) from Tanzania. It seems that young men in Dar es Salaam have incorporated the acronym AIDS into a Kiswahili saying, "*Acha Iniue Dogedego Siachi* (Let it kill me as I will never abandon the young ladies)." This attitude leads to the fatalism voiced by one Tanzanian prostitute, "Even if I take precautions, how can I be completely safe while I have no control over so many things—including my own husband?"

Studies of American adolescents cited in the Citizens Commission report (1989) show continued sexual activity and drug use despite knowledge of modes of HIV transmission. Although there is some evidence that, among 17-to 19-year-old males living in metropolitan areas, condom use is increasing, this is not the case among young men with a history of drug use or of relationships with more than five sexual partners during the past year. Research by the CDC found that 75 percent of graduating high school seniors were sexually active but studies of condom usage have revealed inconsistent behavior by this age group (National Commission on AIDS 1993:7). Public health experts and health educators generally agree that preventive education campaigns are vital in stemming the spread of the epidemic but that they have inherent limitations in achieving short-term behavior change. As Fineberg (1988a:596) remarks, "the evolution of life-style and habit can unfold over a period of decades."

A survey of male homosexuals in an American city demonstrates the difficulty in changing behavior entrenched in life-styles. Although most of the subjects know how AIDS is transmitted and how it may be prevented, they nevertheless think they are taking adequate precautions—although an outside observer might disagree on objective grounds (Ames et al. 1992).

Sociologists Laurie Wermuth, Jennifer Ham, and Rebecca L. Robbins (1992) reviewed the literature on the barriers to behavior change among women partners of drug addicts. A basic premise of prevention messages addressed to women is that, when faced with a noncompliant partner, women will choose not to engage in dangerous and risky behavior. Although seemingly reasonable, this assumption does not take into account the interpersonal, social, and material constraints on such a choice. When individuals do not have equal bargaining power in relationships, the assumption may not apply—particularly in longer term and marital relationships. Social class, gender inequalities, race and ethnicity, and the stigma of being labeled a drug addict all enhance the danger of AIDS among such women.

As an example, the Citizens Commission report (1989) refers to studies of prostitutes showing that they are less likely to use condoms in sexual relations with their boy friends than in commercial transactions with their clients. Some adolescents are at particular risk, the report points out, because of their life-style as homeless wanderers, runaways, prostitutes, teenage partners of homosexual or bisexual men, or drug users. Educational efforts directed at these groups, the report concludes, must be designed to confront the realities of these life-styles.

Keniston (1990) voices a more pessimistic position, seeing sexual behavior and drug use as extremely resistant to educational efforts to change. As evidence, he cites the continuing increase in unwanted pregnancies and the rise in sexually transmitted diseases. In most industrial countries, AIDS is most common among urban populations of young adults "disconnected from formal networks." He believes that optimism concerning education aimed at counteracting intravenous drug use is equally unwarranted, since addiction is still rising despite conventional education campaigns. John Gagnon (1990), a sociologist specializing in the study of sexual behavior, echoes these misgivings, maintaining that it is extremely unlikely that even the most determined education programs can effect major reductions in the number of sexual relationships among the young. He concludes that making behavior change effective is only a hope. But although education to reduce the number of sexual partners may not occur, the use of condoms among the young may make a comeback.

Notwithstanding the many obstacles encountered by efforts in AIDS prevention, Fineberg (1988a:596) concludes that it is crucial to continue "to inform, empower the individual and create a social environment supportive of behavior changes." He notes that "although partial shifts towards safer behaviors will not assure adequate long-term protection to every individual at risk, such changes may nevertheless spell the difference between a serious and a catastrophic epidemic."[5]

The task of changing sexual behavior

Although there is a broad consensus concerning the need to educate the public about how to avoid AIDS, considerably less agreement exists on the ultimate ability of education efforts to mold behavior toward that end. Fineberg (1988a), for example, states that there is now widespread understanding of how to eliminate or greatly reduce the risk for individuals to contract AIDS. By now, the key recommendations—that sexually active men and women should limit their relations to monogamous partnerships, avoid risky sexual practices, or use latex condoms for every episode of intercourse, and that intravenous drugs should be avoided or used only with clean needles without sharing—are by now familiar to an informed public. Thus, the conditions for protecting the nation's health from a dreadful disease exist. Nonetheless, Fineberg sees sex practices and drug use as biologically based and as deriving from impulses that are hard to resist. Although the remarkable change in the behavior of older homosexuals in the United States (reducing the number of partners and the frequency of unprotected anal inter-course) is evidence of the potential effectiveness of AIDS education campaigns, he stresses that long-term protection of an individual requires radical and permanent changes in behavior. Another caveat is that it remains to be seen whether behavior change among the most vulnerable and affected segments of the population can be

---

[5] For a detailed analysis of the needs, problems, and requirements of educating the public about AIDS, see Chapter 2 of National Commission on AIDS (1991c).

effected sufficiently soon to inhibit the spread of the virus. The reduction of HIV transmission among San Francisco homosexuals, for example, brings little comfort when half or more are already infected. In fact, Fineberg is pessimistic about the effect of successful behavior changes on the course of the epidemic in the near term— since those individuals who will develop AIDS in the next few years have already been infected. The best that prevention of virus transmission can achieve, he maintains, is a reduction in cases of clinical disease in the intermediate and long-term future.

Evidence of obstacles encountered in AIDS education is found in a study reported in the *Journal of the American Medical Association* (Zenilman et al. 1992). The research revealed that many patients at an inner-city clinic in Baltimore diagnosed as having been infected with HIV returned within one year with another sexually transmitted disease, despite pre- and post-test counseling to encourage safe sex techniques. The subjects of the study were both male and female; 98 percent were black; and nearly all were heterosexual.

Drawing on the lessons of the history of syphilis, Brandt (1988a) is quite skeptical about the efficacy of education about AIDS. Education that merely expresses fear has limited utility, a fact that is also stressed in the Citizens Commission report (1989). To be effective, education requires a direct confrontation with aspects of sexuality that are typically avoided. Moreover, it is not a panacea for stopping the epidemic, just as it failed to stem other sexually transmitted diseases earlier in the twentieth century. What is needed is greater boldness in the messages as well as careful evaluation of a range of approaches.

For the psychologist Kenneth Keniston, the task of altering behavior in ways that might limit HIV transmission is fraught with enormous difficulties and inherent contradictions. He observes that "every society seeks to control sexual behavior, regulating formally and informally when, with whom, and how sexual relations occur." He adds that "by the same token, every society fails to control sexual behavior completely, and modern societies fail very notably" (1990:xxvi). As evidence, he points to the failure of educational campaigns in industrialized societies designed to prevent unwanted pregnancies. Moreover, AIDS prevention efforts "walk a tightrope between morality and freedom" (xxx). He concludes that

> Morality enters the argument because AIDS is largely
> transmitted through behavior deemed immoral: the
> use of drugs or the practice of extramarital and/or

homosexual sex. But any effective AIDS-prevention strategy must aim at making these "immoral" behaviors safer—by, for example, providing sterile needles and making condoms widely available. Especially in the United States, the desire not to condone "immorality" has effectively prevented the provision of sterile needles and has impeded efforts to provide clear, frank education about safer sex (1990:xxix).

The gap between knowledge and action

Another cause for pessimism concerning the effectiveness of anti-AIDS information campaigns and targeted education efforts is the well-documented gap between knowledge and action, between what people know intellectually and what actions they are willing and capable of taking. As Ehrhardt (1992) maintains, in recent years awareness of how HIV/AIDS is transmitted is relatively high. Moreover, there has been a marked cultural change as reflected in an impressive modification of language and speech: terms such as condom use and anal intercourse, as well as other details of sexual behavior, have become common parlance. "So if people know how HIV and AIDS are transmitted and can talk about it why haven't more people changed their behavior?" Ehrhardt asks (1460).

This gap has many causes. It is a classic concern in behavioral research, and it is the major obstacle in efforts to prevent the spread of the HIV infection. This is a universal problem, being as true of heterosexuals in Africa as of gays in the United States. The failure of information alone to lead to regular and reliable behavior change has been repeatedly documented in varying cultures and contexts. Yet an analysis of the messages in thirty-eight AIDS programs worldwide revealed that, in 90 percent of both industrialized and developing countries, the main messages are simply cautionary (Mann et al. 1992:331).

Sociologists Siegel and Gibson (1988) analyze some of the barriers to behavior modification, including a sense of low personal vulnerability. Another barrier is the selective interpretation of advice concerning methods of risk reduction—for example, restricting the number of partners but also rejecting condoms, which are viewed only as contraceptives. Yet another is confusion about warning messages that contribute to a sense of security among heterosexual men.

Although levels of knowledge about AIDS among young people may be high, survey data show that their behavior does not necessarily reflect it. Despite knowledge of the risk of HIV/STD, a high percentage of 16- to 24-year olds in a cross-national survey conducted in France, the United Kingdom, and the United States continues to engage in high-risk behavior, according to a report presented at the international AIDS conference in Florence in June 1991 (Berezin 1992). The conclusion to be drawn is that education alone does not produce behavioral change; what is required is intervention to change the norms and behavior of close associates, what Berezin calls "social networks." There is evidence, for example, that although education campaigns among addicts led to increased knowledge about AIDS, they did not induce a corresponding change in behavior. In a study of Baltimore addicts, described by Fineberg (1988a:595), knowledge increased significantly although there was no change in needle-sharing behavior. There is evidence, however, that if information about the risks of acquiring HIV infection is combined with the distribution of bleach and with practical instructions for sterilizing intravenous syringes, addicts respond positively. But in general, it has been more difficult to change behavior among drug addicts than among homosexuals. Furthermore, according to data reported by the Citizens Commission, changes in one aspect of behavior are not necessarily followed by other appropriate changes. The report points out that, although some intravenous drug addicts have changed their needle-sharing behavior, they have not changed their sexual behavior to the same degree. And although women and adolescents represent the fastest growing category of new HIV infections, education efforts, which have been extensive, have made little headway.

According to Priscilla R. Ulin (1992), the failure of education campaigns to halt the spread of HIV infection has different causes. Individual strategies for prevention offer narrow options: using condoms and limiting the number and choice of sexual partners. But many women lack the power to negotiate changes in sexual behavior to prevent HIV infection. AIDS prevention campaigns in Africa, she reports, have not taken into account the cultural, social, and economic constraints that limit a woman's ability to comply with such advice as limiting partners and having them use condoms. "For the foreseeable future," Ulin states, "preventing AIDS will continue to depend on the cooperation of both partners. However, until women have it in their power to exercise protection independently, the use of condoms will require women to resort to persuasive or coercive tactics" (63). But this option is difficult because of women's economic dependency and the social expectation that she will play a compliant female role.[6]

Citing Worth's research, Ulin notes that women in New York City have invested condoms with socially conditioned meanings that often bar their use. For example, condoms are viewed as evidence of a desire to have unnatural sex. In sub-Saharan Africa, condoms are associated with contraception, and the limited success of family planning programs in this region illustrates the limitations of their use in AIDS prevention. The resistance of African families to contraception, Ulin says, has hindered efforts to prevent perinatal HIV infection among women in Zaire. Men and women share the burden of AIDS and the responsibility for preventing it, but AIDS prevention messages have a different impact on men and women. The key to the modification of behavior, Ulin asserts, requires a "delicate balance of decision making" (71).

Ehrhardt (1992) also criticizes the messages directed at women, calling them simplistic and not grounded in the realities of women's lives or in aspects of their life that are under their control. For example, for women to protect themselves by having their partner use condoms, the message should be directed to heterosexual men. Moreover, women in America today are on average single for many years before their first marriage; they might be single again after a divorce; they might marry again; and ultimately they might be widowed. For some women, multiple partners throughout their life is an economic necessity. Thus, exhortations to reduce the number of partners are meaningless unless a woman's economic status improves.

The Need for Research on Sexual Behavior

In most of the world's epidemics, the core activity in the transmission of HIV infection is sexual behavior. Yet, more than any previous epidemic, AIDS has illustrated the complexity of the task of changing behavior that is rooted in biology, in individual psychological needs, in social class, and in culture. As Misztal and Moss (1990:9) point out, "in all societies, the dimensions, forms, and social distribution of sexual preferences and activity remain almost totally uncharted." Ironically, in the United States, which has a

---

[6] Ulin remarks that one reported unintended consequence of AIDS information campaigns in Zaire is that some men are beginning to leave the older sex workers in favor of young schoolgirls who, they reason, are unlikely to be infected with HIV.

strong tradition of social research, large sums of money available for research, and a considerable toleration of public discussions of sexual behavior, less is known about prevailing patterns of sexual behavior than about AIDS itself.   As Ehrhardt (1992) notes, a fundamental problem is that educational messages have been designed without systematic and detailed information about people's sexual behavior. Research on sexual behavior has been sporadic and incomplete, difficult to fund, and vulnerable to objections from many quarters to investigations of this most private behavior. In spite of these many obstacles, some useful research has been carried out.[7]

In an editorial in the *Journal of the American Medical Association*, James R. Allen and Valerie P. Setlow (1991) outline an agenda for urgently needed cross-cultural social research. They point out that the most common risk factors for HIV infection were isolated a decade ago and were used to identify and describe epidemic patterns in different areas and countries. But these "broad brush strokes" make it difficult to understand the subtle complexities of HIV transmission in different geographical areas and subgroups. Citing two studies of sexual behavior, one in Rwanda and one in California, which compare the risk factors in sexual relations that are constant in both cultures, the authors stress the need for additional studies that will help identify the high-risk behaviors of different people in different geographical areas and population groups.

We need better information about why people make the choices they do, Allen and Setlow maintain. We need to know what information they have about HIV infection that might influence these choices and how physicians, health educators, public health officials, the school system, community organizations, and others can provide effective education. Finally, based on the information from these studies, we must try to develop more effective prevention programs, considering not only infection transmission patterns but also prevailing sexual standards and practices. Failure to do this in the United States and elsewhere will ensure continued transmission of HIV.

The efficacy of education on condom use was examined in a nationwide study reported in *Science* (Catania et al. 1992). The researchers interviewed by telephone a national sample of 10,630

---

[7] For a review of relevant research published in the 1980s, see Levy and Albrecht (1989).

adults composed of two groups: a national sample and a sample of people living in high-risk cities. The purpose of the study was to assess the prevalence of HIV-related risk factors (e.g., having sex with multiple partners or with partners themselves at risk) among the general heterosexual population. The study found that condom use is relatively low, but that young people in their twenties, who have been major targets of education campaigns, are to some extent responding to messages about them. But sexually active middle-aged and older adults have not been reached. In all, 70 percent of the high-risk takers never use condoms. The researchers conclude that "it remains to be seen whether the apparent lack of concern by heterosexuals for the risks associated with STDs will change as a result of media attention given to public figures such as Earvin 'Magic' Johnson" (1105).[8] (See Chapter 3 for other details of this study.)

The National Commission on AIDS, in its 1991 report, urged that higher priority and increased funding should be given to social, behavioral, and health services research. At the eighth international conference on AIDS in Amsterdam in 1992, the participants called for the development of valid and practical methods for measuring behavioral change (Bryce 1992).

The Gagnon research agenda

Notwithstanding a strong tradition of research on human behavior in the United States, sex has been a much neglected topic of research: less is known about the motivations, the variety of expressions, and the prevalence among subgroups of the population of this activity than of any other. Surveys of sexual behavior based on national representative samples have been difficult to fund, encountering both political opposition and public reticence.

Social scientists have long recognized the need to learn more about the prevalence of various forms of sexual behavior throughout the population and how it varies with age and ethnicity. The sociologist John H. Gagnon (1990) has provided an overview of this kind of fundamental research, focusing specifically on sexual behavior that is crucial to understanding the social dimensions of the U.S. AIDS epidemic. He stresses that an epidemiological picture of AIDS in the immediate and middle range future depends on

---

8 For additional discussion of the impact of AIDS prevention messages on sexual behavior, see Hardy and Biddlecom (1991) and Biddlecom and Hardy (1991).

acquiring more substantive knowledge of (1) what people do in the privacy of their bedrooms or in other places; (2) the social networks of sexually defined subgroups, such as homosexuals; (3) the dynamics of the subculture of adolescents and young adults before marriage; (4) the largely hidden phenomenon of bisexuality; and (5) the dominant patterns of sexual behavior among heterosexuals.

Gagnon believes that the AIDS crisis has engendered a particular need for research on sexuality in the following areas. Unless otherwise indicated, this section is based on his 1990 essay, "Disease and Desire."

Homosexual life styles. The homosexual community, reacting to the threat and reality of AIDS, has encouraged a conception of a loving, stable life-style that replaces the indiscriminate sexual "cruising" that was practiced in the 1970s and early 1980s. What is not known is how pervasive this life-style is in gay communities or whether it is found among young persons just entering gay life.

Data are also needed on homosexual behavior in minority and working-class communities. Thus far, research has focused on white, male, moderately well-educated gay communities. "Everyone and everywhere else," says Gagnon, is "*terra obscura*" (1990:188).

Bisexuality. With the advent of AIDS, bisexual men are seen as constituting a potential "bridge" for infection to cross from the gay to the heterosexual world. Bisexuality, Gagnon believes, represents a serious scientific problem for research driven by the AIDS epidemic; it resists being easily categorized.

The role of drugs in sexual behavior. The AIDS epidemic has focused attention on the sexual behavior of illicit drug users, on their needle-sharing behavior, and on the exchange of sex for crack. Systematic research is needed to explore the nature and extent of these patterns of behavior as well as the use of crack and cocaine as aphrodisiacs.

Heterosexual behavior. Heterosexual behavior has many manifestations that vary in different social strata; it is influenced by class, race, ethnicity, marital status, religion, and education. The epidemic has posed its own questions about the structure of social relations among the heterosexual majority. Who has sex with whom, the number of sexual partners, the differences that sex-for-pay make, and relationships with one-time casual partners—in short, how sexual life is organized—are examples of the questions that need to be asked.

Sexual behavior of the young. The young are influenced more by each other and by the sexual practices of their peers than they are by what adults tell them. However, the purpose of much current research on sexuality among young people is to assess their conduct and evaluate the impact of educational programs. Most studies do not attempt to trace the relevant processes of psychosexual development or to determine how sexuality became such an important part of the lives of young Americans.

The NORC study

In response to a call for proposals from the National Institute of Child Health and Human Development, the National Opinion Research Center (NORC), a social science research center at the University of Chicago, proposed in 1987 that a nationwide representative sample survey on sexual behavior be undertaken. The NORC proposal (1987) noted that changing patterns of sexual conduct as well as demographic shifts in the composition of the U.S. population have led, during recent years, to startling increases not only in AIDS but also in other "traditional" sexually transmitted diseases (syphilis, gonorrhea) and "new" diseases such as herpes, papilloma, and chlamydia as well. The data on sexual behavior necessary to cope with this changing situation in American society are sparse. Sexuality, the proposal stated, has rarely been a topic considered suitable for scientific analysis or reasoned public discussion.

The bulk of research on sexuality extending from the time of Freud to that of the biologist Alfred C. Kinsey was mainly clinical or criminological in orientation. The Kinsey studies, the first of which was published in 1948 and which surveyed a large number of individuals on their sexual behavior, are the basis for much of what is known or thought to be known today about sexual behavior in the United States. The Kinsey studies, however, were not based on samples representative of the population as a whole. Rather, they were based on self-reports by individuals, most of whom were recruited for the study by one of the institutions cooperating with the researchers. In more recent years, several studies of sexual attitudes and behavior, also based on "convenience" rather than representative samples, were undertaken by popular magazines (*McCalls, Playboy, Redbook*), but they have been methodologically flawed and are not considered to be reliable sources of information.

The proposal went through several favorable reviews by government agencies. In the Congress, conservative opponents of the research characterized the questionnaire they reviewed as pornographic—presumably because it employed line drawings and other visual devices in order to ask people how many sexual partners they had had, what sort of acts they performed with them, and what their views were of what they did.

Proponents of the study, including major social scientists advising the National Research Council, maintained that this kind of information on sexual practices is vital for predicting and mitigating the spread of AIDS. The proposal was sent to Secretary of Health and Human Services Louis Sullivan. who supported the intent of the study but found problems with the tone and content of the questions used in the survey instrument (*Science*, Research News, April 8, 1990). Approval of this research was withheld until April 2, 1992, when, by an overwhelming vote of 87–10, the Senate passed the National Institutes of Health Reauthorization Bill which included provisions allowing federally funded surveys of human sexual behavior. There had been a similar vote in the House in July 1991 (*COSSA Washington Update*, April 6, 1992:1); accordingly, objections to the study were apparently removed.

In the meantime, NORC had undertaken a massive and successful fund-raising campaign among private foundations and had obtained support from seven, including the American Foundation for AIDS Research, for a somewhat scaled-down version of the original study plan. A national sample of 3,200 persons was studied through personal interviews. The field work was finished in August 1992, and the analysis was carried out in the winter and spring of 1993 (Lyon 1992; NORC 1992).

The Battelle studies

In 1993, the results of the National Survey of Men, carried out by a team of social scientists at the Battelle Human Affairs Research Center, Seattle, Washington, were published in the March/April issue of *Family Planning Perspectives*. The survey is one of the first representative surveys of the sexual behavior of U.S. men. As an editorial in the journal by Olivia Schieffelin Nordberg points out (1993), most previous surveys have used "convenience" or other nonrepresentative samples: the National Survey of Men is "in a category by itself." She notes that the survey provides data on what proportion of men have engaged in vaginal, anal, and oral sex and whether differences in sexual behavior exist in various relationships such as marriage, cohabitation, and steady partnerships (Billy et al. 1993). It analyzes what kinds of men are most likely to use condoms and whether the color and design of condoms are deemed important (Tanfer et al. 1993; Grady et al 1993). And it reports how perceptions of the risk and severity of AIDS affects sexual behavior (Klepinger et al. 1993).

Valuable as these new data are, they do not provide information on the scale deemed necessary to provide fully comprehensive knowledge of male sexual behavior; researchers would like to see surveys of 10 to 25 thousand people. But the costs of such surveys ($15 to 20 million) are likely to deter any such proposal (Watson 1993).

The National Research Council reviews

Two major reports by teams of social scientists acknowledge the complexity of the task of changing both social and sexual behavior. Their findings show that designing effective change strategies urgently requires social research on (1) patterns of sexual behavior among populations at risk; (2) the efficacy of various prevention strategies, such as counseling and condom distribution; and (3) the efficacy of education efforts aimed at different groups.

With funds from the Centers for Disease Control, the National Research Council (NRC)—the research arm of the National Academy of Sciences—appointed a Committee on AIDS Research and the Behavioral, Social, and Statistical Research, chaired by Lincoln E. Moses, a statistician at Stanford University. The committee's major publications include *AIDS: Sexual Behavior and Intravenous Drug Use* (Turner et al. 1989) and *AIDS: The Second Decade* (Miller et al. 1990). [A third publication, *The Social Impact of AIDS in the United States* (Jonsen & Stryker 1993) is reviewed in Chapter 3.]

The first two NRC publications are essentially reviews of existing research reports and outlines of social research that needs to be carried out. Three questions are addressed:

1. How many Americans are infected with HIV, and what are their characteristics?
2. How can transmission be stopped?
3. How do we know that public health intervention is working?

In the conclusion of *AIDS: Sexual Behavior and Intravenous Drug Use* (Turner et al. 1989), the editors set forth two broad propositions: (1) AIDS has forced American society to examine itself and (2) knowledge of sexual behavior is central to an understanding of the epidemic. Yet current knowledge of patterns of sexual behavior is fragmentary and unreliable. Consequently, attempts to contain what is essentially a sexually transmitted disease (STD) epidemic through education and other intervention strategies—without adequate knowledge of the behavior that spreads the disease—are severely hobbled.[9]

The editors recommend a vigorous program of basic social and behavioral research on human sexual behavior, conducted through a consortium of governmental health research agencies. If AIDS prevention programs are to be targeted more effectively, more must be known about who is at risk. What is needed is research on the prevalence of risk-taking behaviors in various populations—including both low- and high-risk groups. Because sexual behavior is influenced by cultural norms and values, the social context of the behavior must be studied. Because sexual behavior is dynamic—evolving and changing through the life course—the authors stress the need for longitudinal studies (that is, studies of the same sample of individuals at different points in time). Understanding the behavior of high-risk groups such as prostitutes and their clients, gays who live outside of major population centers, drug and alcohol abusers, and certain adolescents is also essential. The editors stress that the country is now paying the costs that result when prospective studies are interrupted and research programs are subject to feast-or-famine cycles of support—a clear reference to criticism of research on sexual behavior made by members of the Congress.

The NRC's second report, *AIDS: The Second Decade* (Miller et al. 1990), reaffirms the importance of behavioral change as the primary weapon against AIDS. Addressing the problem of the danger of HIV infections to adolescents, the editors stress that there is some evidence that STDs are a greater problem in younger populations than in older ones. Yet little is known about adolescent sexual behavior; for example, about homosexual experimentation, about anal intercourse, and about other risky sexual practices—although there is evidence that these behaviors occur. Furthermore, continued risk taking does not appear to be related to unawareness of the threat posed by unprotected sexual contacts. As long as sexual behavior that promotes HIV infection exists in the adolescent population, it is imperative to learn about it, to note the populations and geographic areas in which the risky behaviors tend to occur,

---

[9] The National Commission on AIDS has pointed out that, although teenagers are urged in some educational campaigns to delay sexual intercourse until marriage or adulthood, a majority of young people has not heeded this advice, no matter how forcefully the message is delivered (National Commission on AIDS 1992b).

and to direct intervention resources toward those areas to prevent AIDS.

An added dividend from this research is that it will suggest ways of coping with other long-standing problems of adolescence such as STDs and unintended pregnancies. The specific role of drug use both in spreading HIV infection through needle sharing and in encouraging risky sexual behavior is another crucial area of research. The editors maintain that national surveys of drug users that include teenagers are nonetheless likely to underestimate the size of the problem among them. School-based surveys among high school students do not capture dropouts or chronic absentees, and individuals omitted from both household and school-based surveys are known to have higher rates of drug use than does the general population. It is therefore necessary to conduct research among adolescents that will enable public health authorities to intervene before the syndrome of risky sexual and drug-use behavior begins. Finally, evaluation research must be conducted to assess the effectiveness of various intervention programs.[10]

Prevention through Education

More than any previous epidemic, AIDS has illustrated the complexity of the task of changing behavior through education. The problem is compounded by the fact that there is considerable dissension and doubt in the international community of specialists concerned with the task of prevention through education. In its opening statement, the fourth meeting of the Institute of Medicine's International Forum for AIDS Research noted that

> Behavioral interventions for the prevention of sexual transmission of HIV infections, although frequently discussed and adopted, are little understood. For some,

---

[10] The lack of research on sexual behavior is not unique to the United States. In France, despite the liberalization of sexual mores in the 1960s, very little research has been done on sexuality (D'Aubigny et al. 1990), although a large-scale study financed by the French government was reported on in 1992 (*New York Times*, December 8, 1992:C3). Prime Minister Thatcher canceled a national survey of sexual attitudes and behavior in the United Kingdom by denying government funding—because of her distaste for intrusion into privacy (Street & Weale 1992). The study was subsequently undertaken with private funding from the Wellcome Trust.

they are crucial for the present and for the foreseeable future because they are the only strategy at hand until tested preventive and curative therapies become readily available. For others, the concept is too nebulous and elusive to operationalize or assess. And for many, the changing of human behavior in any durable, consistent way is simply impossible. A further impediment to understanding behavioral interventions is the rich diversity of disciplines involved, each with its own language and distinctive approach. The net effect is some considerable confusion, not a little skepticism, and what amounts to a schism between the biomedical and social scientific communities. While that schism is not new, it is, in the case of the HIV infections, particularly unproductive (Institute of Medicine 1991:1).

The forum's major methodological contribution was the development of a model for classifying and studying different behavioral interventions designed to prevent HIV transmission:

1. "Strategies targeted to the individual" means AIDS prevention counseling, either in groups or in one-on-one interaction.
2. "Strategies targeted to the community" means the use both of local mass media and existing social networks.
3. "Strategies targeted across communities" means the use of radio and television on a national or an international level.

One allegedly successful tactic was reported at a U.S. Department of State press conference (*New York Times*, November 28, 1991:B15). Jeff Harris, director of the AIDS program for USAID, reported that in developing countries where the use of condoms is vigorously promoted, they have been accepted. Marketing techniques, based on marketing research, using television advertising, have successfully promoted condoms in such areas as the Caribbean, the Dominican Republic, Equador, Mexico, and Turkey. "We market condoms the way we would Coca Cola," Harris said.

Clearly, permanent behavior change that will survive transient fads and appeals and that will affect succeeding generations must be firmly based in cultural acceptance. As many observers have noted, many messages urging the use of condoms and the reduction in the number of sexual encounters are directed at women, but without a true understanding of the facts of women's lives and their subordinate role in sexual relations. In the myriad subcultures of sub-Saharan Africa, which remains the epicenter of the pandemic, the task is made even more difficult by different cultural definitions of sex. The Africanist Robert J. Earickson believes that there is an even deeper reason: the message of AIDS, like that of other cultural imports, is one that is derived from the West. It is, he says

> A foreign concept in a foreign language that is dependent on the West for its meaning and continued development. It speaks in Western metaphors and with a voice that was born from that cultural cosmology. It is not indigenous to the Third World and thus is blind to their world of meaning (Earickson 1990:960).

Of course, many in the West think that AIDS is not indigenous to their world either. In an article entitled "Overcoming Denial," Elliot Aronson et al. (1991) point out that surveys reveal that most young adults believe that AIDS is a serious problem, but they have trouble believing that it is *their* problem. If they have convinced themselves that they are not at risk, why should they change their behavior?

This review of efforts both in the United States and abroad to change the behavior of people who are at risk of HIV infection in ways that will decrease that risk contains very few success stories. In the United States, which has a large profession of public health educators and a record of some successes, the difficulty seems to be in deflecting the motivations that lead to both sexual intercourse and drug use. These are powerful motivations, and the history of controlling both traditional sexually transmitted diseases and the use of illicit drugs is for the most part largely one of great frustration.

The phrase "education and prevention" is perhaps the major talisman invoked by AIDS workers throughout the world; until a vaccine and a cure are found, it is said repeatedly, the only hope is to change individual behavior. The limits to changing sexual behavior through massive AIDS education programs aimed primarily at individuals were described by the public health historian Stephen B. Thomas in testimony before the National Commission on AIDS on June 15, 1992. He noted that during the first decade of AIDS the focus of public health efforts was almost entirely on interrupting the cycle of HIV transmission. The assumption was that the targets of information campaigns were educated people eager to do the right thing if only they had the appropriate information. He concluded that this definition of the task is inadequate:

> We cannot expect a national education campaign based only on information alone to change recalcitrant problems. The spread of HIV has highlighted the complex relationship among social class, gender, and race in a society where health care facilities are impoverished, access to care is inadequate, and prevention technology is devalued (quoted in National Commission on AIDS 1992b:12).

To say that poverty must be reduced, that health care services must be improved, and that such items of prevention technology as condoms must be more highly valued is not tantamount to exonerating individuals for the transmission of HIV or to say that society must correct its failures if AIDS is to be conquered. Rather, it is to say that individuals behave in a social, cultural, and economic context that is not of their making, and that efforts to reach them must be accompanied by efforts to reform or revolutionize the communities and the societies in which they live.

AIDS is caused by a virus, but the disease is the result of human behavior that transmits the vector, HIV. The "enemy" that activates the virus is human behavior—at truck stops and in the barracks of migrant workers, in the thatched huts of rural villages, in the slum shanties of the developing world, in the bedrooms of the inner-city poor, in the hotel rooms and large houses of the not-so-poor, in houses of prostitution, and in big-city bathhouses. This behavior is driven by culture, by ignorance, by despair, by desire, and by love—and of course by the age-old male domination of women. To change it is the challenge of our times.

References

AIDS: An Opportunity Not to Be Lost. 1992. *The Lancet* 340 (July 18):147–148.

Aiken, Jane Harris. 1987. "Education as Prevention." In *AIDS and the Law*, edited by Harlon L. Dalton et al. New Haven, Conn.: Yale Univ. Press.

Alden, John S., et al. 1991. *Managing Uganda's Orphan Crisis.* Washington, D.C.: U.S. Agency for International Development.

Allen, James R., and Valerie P. Setlow. 1991. Heterosexual Transmission of HIV: A View of the Future. *Journal of the American Medical Association* 266 (September 25):1695–1696.

Altman, Dennis. 1986. *AIDS in the Mind of America.* Garden City, N. Y.: Doubleday.

Altman, Dennis. 1988. "Legitimization through Disaster: AIDS and the Gay Movement." In *AIDS: The Burdens of History*, edited by Elizabeth Fee and Daniel M. Fox. Berkeley: Univ. of California Press.

Altman, Dennis. 1990. AIDS and Homosexual Groups: Southeast Asia. *AIDS & Society* (April):6.

Altman, Dennis. 1991. Australia: A Partnership against AIDS. *AIDS & Society* (April/May):10.

Altman, Dennis. 1992. "Dehomosexualization." In *AIDS in the World*, edited by Jonathan Mann et al., 388–389. Cambridge, Mass.: Harvard Univ. Press.

Altman, Dennis. 1993. Conference Opinion: Amsterdam. *AIDS & Society* (January/February):7.

American Academy of Orthopaedic Surgeons. 1991. "Advisory

Statement on HIV-infected Orthopaedic Surgeons." March. Park Ridge, Ill: The Academy.

American Medical Association. 1991. "AMA Statement on HIV-infected Physicians." January 17. Chicago: The Association.

American Sociological Association. 1991. *The Sociology of AIDS: Six Lectures and Materials for Instructors and Students.* Washington, D.C.: The Association.

Ames, Lynda J., et al. 1992. "Love, Lust, Fear: Safer Sex Decision Making among Gay Men." Unpublished paper. Department of Sociology, State University of New York, Plattsburgh, N.Y.

Anastos, Kathryn, and Carola Marte. 1991. "Women—The Missing Persons in the AIDS Epidemic." In *The AIDS Reader,* edited by Nancy F. McKenzie. New York: Meridian.

Anderson, R. M., et al. 1991. The Spread of HIV-1 in Africa: Sexual Contact Patterns and the Predicted Demographic Impact of AIDS. *Nature* 352 (August 15):581–589.

Armtrong, Jill. 1991. Socioeconomic Implications of AIDS in Developing Countries. *Finance & Development* (December):14–17.

Armstrong, Jill, and Eduard Bos. 1992. "The Demographic, Economic, and Social Impact of AIDS." In *AIDS in the World,* edited by Jonathan Mann et al., 195–226. Cambridge, Mass.: Harvard Univ. Press.

Arno, Peter. 1991. "Housing, Homelessness, and the Impact of HIV Disease." In *The AIDS Reader,* edited by Nancy F. McKenzie. New York: Meridian.

Arnow, Paul M., et al. 1989. Orthopedic Surgeons' Attitudes and Practices Concerning Treatment of Patients with HIV Infection. *Public Health Reports* 104 (March/April):121–129.

Aronson, Elliot, et al. 1991. Overcoming Denial and Increasing the Intention to Use Condoms through the Induction of Hypocrisy. *American Journal of Public Health* 81 (December):1636-1641.

Baker, Andrea J. 1986. "The Portrayal of AIDS in the Media: An Analysis of Articles in the New York Times." In *Social Dimensions of AIDS,* edited by Douglas A. Feldman and Thomas M. Johnson. New York: Praeger.

Barnett, Tony, and Piers Blaikie. 1992. *AIDS in Africa: Its Present and Future Impact.* New York: Guilford Press.

Bartlett, Lawrence. 1990. "Financing Health Care for Persons with AIDS: Balancing Public and Private Responsibilities." In *AIDS and the Health Care System,* edited by Lawrence O. Gostin. New Haven, Conn.: Yale Univ. Press.

Bayer, Ronald. 1989. *Private Acts, Social Consequences: AIDS and the Politics of Public Health.* New York: Free Press.

Bayer, Ronald. 1991a. AIDS: The Politics of Prevention and Neglect. *Health Affairs* (Spring):87–97.

Bayer, Ronald. 1991b. "AIDS, Public Health and Civil Liberties: Consensus and Conflict in Policy." In *AIDS & Ethics,* edited by Frederic G. Reamer. New York: Columbia Univ. Press.

Bayer, Ronald. 1992. "Entering the Second Decade: The Politics of Prevention, the Politics of Neglect." In *AIDS: The Making of a Chronic Disease,* edited by Elizabeth Fee and Daniel M. Fox. Berkeley: Univ. of California Press.

Bazell, Robert. 1992. Happy Campers. *New Republic* (March 9):12–14.

Becker, Charles M. 1990. The Demo-Economic Impact of the AIDS Pandemic on Sub-Saharan Africa. *World Development* 18 (12):1599–1619.

Becker, Marshall H., and Jill D. Joseph. 1988. AIDS and Behavioral Change to Reduce Risk. *American Journal of Public Health* 78 (April):394–410.

Beer, Christopher, et al. 1988. "AIDS—The Grandmother's Burden." In *The Global Impact of AIDS,* edited by Alan F. Fleming et al. New York: Alan R. Liss.

Bell, David M. 1990. "HIV Infection in Health Care Workers: Occupational Risk and Infection." In *AIDS and the Health Care System,* edited by Lawrence O. Gostin. New Haven, Conn.: Yale Univ. Press.

Berezin, Nancy. 1992. "HIV and Other Sexually Transmitted Diseases." In *AIDS in the World,* edited by Jonathan Mann et al., 165–193. Cambridge, Mass.: Harvard Univ. Press.

Berk, Richard A., ed. 1988. *The Social Impact of AIDS in the U. S.* Cambridge, Mass.: Abt Books.

Berkley, Seth. 1992. Amsterdam Viewpoint: Costly Regional AIDS Conference for the North. *AIDS & Society* (July/August):3–4.

Biddlecom, Ann E., and Ann M. Hardy. 1991. "AIDS Knowledge and Attitudes of Hispanic Americans: United States, 1990." A report of the National Center for Health Statistics. Hyattsville, Md.: The Center.

Billy, John O. G., et al. 1993. The Sexual Behavior of Men in the United States. *Family Planning Perspectives* 25(March/April):52–60.

Blendon, Robert J., and Karen Donelan. 1989. "AIDS, the Public, and the 'NIMBY' Syndrome." In *Public and Professional Atti-*

tudes toward AIDS Patients, edited by David E. Rogers and Eli Ginzburg. Boulder, Colo.: Westview Press.

Blendon, Robert J., and Karen Donelan. 1990. "AIDS and Discrimination: Public and Professional Perspectives." In *AIDS and the Health Care System,* edited by Lawrence O. Gostin. New Haven, Conn.: Yale Univ. Press.

Bloom, David E., and Geoffrey Carliner. 1988. "The Economic Impact of AIDS in the United States." In *AIDS 1988,* edited by Ruth Kulstad. Washington, D.C.: American Association for the Advancement of Science.

Blumberg, Baruch S. 1988. Hepatitis B Virus and the Carrier Problem. *Social Research* 55 (3):401-412.

Bongaarts, John, and Peter Way. 1989. "Geographic Variation in the HIV Epidemic and the Impact of AIDS in Africa." The Population Council, Research Division, *Working Papers,* No. 1. New York: The Council.

Bongaarts, John, et al. 1989. The Relationship between Male Circumcision and HIV Infection in African Populations. *AIDS* 3 (June):373–377.

Bosk, Charles, and Joel E. Frader. 1991. "AIDS and Its Impact on Medical Work: The Culture and Politics of the Shop Floor." In *A Disease of Society,* edited by Dorothy Nelkin et al. New York: Cambridge Univ. Press.

Brandt, Allan M. 1987. *No Magic Bullet: A Social History of Venereal Disease in the United States since 1880.* New York: Oxford Univ. Press.

Brandt, Allan M. 1988a. AIDS in Historical Perspective: Four Lessons from the History of Sexually Transmitted Diseases. *American Journal of Public Health* 78 (April):367–371.

Brandt, Allan M. 1988b. AIDS and Metaphor: Toward the Social Meaning of Epidemic Disease. *Social Research* 55 (3):413–432.

Brandt, Allan M. 1988c. "From Social History to Social Policy." In *AIDS: The Burdens of History,* edited by Elizabeth Fee and Daniel M. Fox. Berkeley: Univ. of California Press.

Brandt, Allan M. 1988d. The Syphilis Epidemic and Its Relation to AIDS. *Science* 239 (January 22):375380.

Brennan, Troyen A. 1990. "Occupational Transmission of HIV: An Ethical and Legal Challenge." In *AIDS and the Health Care System,* edited by Lawrence O. Gostin. New Haven, Conn.: Yale Univ. Press.

Bresolin, L. B., et al. 1990. Attitudes of U.S. Primary Care Physicians about HIV Disease and AIDS. *AIDS Care* 2 (2):117125.

Brookmeyer, Ron. 1991. Reconstruction and Future Trends of the AIDS Epidemic in the United States. *Science* 253 (July 5):3742.

Brown, Arthur. 1988. "AIDS—Impact on Development Programmes." Unpublished paper delivered at the Fourth International Conference on AIDS, Stockholm. Abstract No. 9608. June 13–14.

Brown, Phyllida. 1992. "AIDS in the Media." In *AIDS in the World*, edited by Jonathan Mann et al., 720–732. Cambridge, Mass.: Harvard Univ. Press.

Bryce, Jennifer. 1992. "Amsterdam Report: Issues of Social Impact and Response." *AIDS & Society* (July/August):5, 8.

Buehler, James W. 1992a. The Reporting of HIV/AIDS Deaths in Women. *American Journal of Public Health* 82 (November):15001505.

Buehler, James W. 1992b. The Surveillance Definition for AIDS. *American Journal of Public Health* 82 (November):1462–1464.

Caldwell, John C., et al. 1989. The Social Context of AIDS in Sub-Saharan Africa. *Population and Development Review* (June):185–234.

Cameron, Charles. 1992. "Providing Care." In *AIDS in the World*, edited by Jonathan Mann et al., 449–475. Cambridge, Mass.: Harvard Univ. Press.

Caplan, Pat, ed. 1988. *The Cultural Construction of Sexuality*. London: Tavistock Publications.

Carballo, M., and M. Carael. 1988. "Impact of AIDS on Social Organization." In *The Global Impact of AIDS*, edited by Alan F. Fleming et al. New York: Alan R. Liss.

Carovano, Kathryn. 1987. "AIDS and Poverty in the Third World." Overseas Development Council, *Policy Focus* 7 (October):1–10.

Catania, Joseph A., et al. 1992. Prevalence of AIDS-related Risk Factors and Condom Use in the United States. *Science* 258 (November 13):1101–1106.

Chin, James. 1988. "HIV and International Travel." In *The Global Impact of AIDS*, edited by Alan F. Fleming et al. New York: Alan R. Liss.

Chirimuuta, Richard, et al. 1988. "The Spread of Racism." In *The AIDS Reader*, edited by Loren K. Clarke and Malcolm Potts. Boston: Brandon Publishing Co.

Chitwood, Dale D., et al. 1991. The Donation and Sale of Blood by Intravenous Drug Users. *American Journal of Public Health* 81 (May):631–633.

Christakis, Nicholas A. 1990. "Responding to a Pandemic: International Interests in AIDS Control." In *Living with AIDS*, edited by Stephen R. Graubard. Cambridge, Mass.: MIT Press.

Citizens Commission on AIDS for New York and Northern New Jersey. 1988. *AIDS and Drug Use: Breaking the Link.* September. New York: The Commission.

Citizens Commission on AIDS for New York and Northern New Jersey. 1989. *AIDS Prevention and Education: Reframing the Message.* November. New York: The Commission.

Citizens Commission on AIDS for New York and Northern New Jersey. 1991. *Is There a Will to Meet the Challenge?* February. New York: The Commission.

Clarke, Loren K., and Malcolm Potts, eds. 1988a. *The AIDS Reader: Documentary History of a Modern Epidemic.* Boston: Brandon Publishing Co.

Clarke, Loren K., and Malcolm Potts. 1988b. "The Spread of Racism." In *The AIDS Reader,* edited by Loren K. Clarke and Malcolm Potts. Boston: Brandon Publishing Co.

Clarke, Oscar W., and Robert B. Conley. 1991. The Duty to "Attend upon the Sick." *Journal of the American Medical Association* 266 (November 27):2876–2877.

Clayton, Alastair J. 1989. "Building a New Perspective on AIDS." Interview in *AIDS '89 Bulletin.* Fifth International Conference on AIDS, Montreal. June 49.

Colasanto, Diane, et al. 1992. Context Effects on Responses to Questions about AIDS. *Public Opinion Quarterly* 56 (Winter):515–518.

Colombotos, John, et al. 1991. "Physicians, Nurses and AIDS: Preliminary Findings from a National Study." Unpublished paper, Columbia University School of Public Health, Division of Sociomedical Sciences. June 12.

Conant, Francis Paine. 1988. "Social Consequences of AIDS: Implications for East Africa and the Eastern United States." In *AIDS 1988,* edited by Ruth Kulstad. Washington, D.C.: American Association for the Advancement of Science.

Condit, Douglas, and Robert W. M. Frater. 1988. "Human Immunodeficiency Virus and the Cardiac Surgeon: A Survey of Attitudes." Unpublished paper delivered at the 24th annual meeting of the Society of Thoracic Surgeons, New Orleans, Louisiana.

Conference Opinion: Amsterdam. 1993. *AIDS & Society* (January/February):7.

Cook, Timothy E., and David C. Colby. 1992. "The Mass-mediated Epidemic: The Politics of AIDS on the Nightly Network News." In *AIDS: The Making of a Chronic Disease*, edited by Elizabeth Fee and Daniel M. Fox. Berkeley: Univ. of California Press.

Cordeiro, Hesio. 1988. "Medical Costs of HIV and AIDS in Brazil." In *The Global Impact of AIDS*, edited by Alan F. Fleming et al. New York: Alan R. Liss.

Corless, Inge B., and Mary Pittman-Lindeman, eds. 1988. *AIDS: Principles, Practices, & Politics*. Washington, D.C.: Hemisphere Publishing Corp.

Cotton, Deborah J. 1988. "The Impact of AIDS on the Medical Care System." In *AIDS 1988*, edited by Ruth Kulstad. Washington, D.C.: American Association for the Advancement of Science.

Craven, Donald E. 1988. "AIDS in Intravenous Drug Users." In *AIDS 1988*, edited by Ruth Kulstad. Washington, D.C.: American Association for the Advancement of Science.

Craven, Donald E. 1989. " Human Immunodeficiency Virus in Intravenous Drug Users: Epidemiology, Issues, and Controversies." In *The AIDS Epidemic*, edited by Padraig O'Malley. Boston: Beacon Press.

Crosby, Alfred W. 1989. *America's Forgotten Pandemic: The Influenza of 1918*. New York: Cambridge Univ. Press. [First published in 1976 as *Epidemic and Peace: 1918*.]

Crystal, Stephen, and Marguerite Jackson. 1992. "Health Care and the Social Construction of AIDS: The Impact of Disease Definition." In *The Social Context of AIDS*, edited by Joan Huber and Beth E. Schneider. Beverly Hills, Calif.: Sage Publications.

Crystal, Stephen, et al. 1989. "Persons with AIDS and Older People: Common Long-term Care Concerns." In *AIDS in an Aging Society*, edited by Matilda White Riley et al. New York: Springer.

Curran, James W., et al. 1988. "Epidemiology of AIDS and HIV Infection in the United States." In *AIDS 1988*, edited by Ruth Kulstad. Washington, D.C.: American Association for the Advancement of Science.

Dalton, Harlon L. 1990. "AIDS in Blackface." In *Living with AIDS*, edited by Stephen R. Graubard. Cambridge, Mass.: MIT Press.

Dalton, Harlon L., et al., eds. 1987. *AIDS and the Law: A Guide for the Public*. New Haven, Conn.: Yale Univ. Press.

Darrow, William W., et al. 1988. "Behaviors Associated with HIV-1 Infection and the Development of AIDS." In *AIDS 1988*, edited by Ruth Kulstad. Washington, D.C.: American Association for the Advancement of Science.

D'Aubigny, Gérard, et al. 1990. SIDA, comportements sexuels et attitudes sociales. *Revue Française des Affaires Sociales* (October):97–107.

Dearing, James W. 1992. "Foreign Blood and Domestic Politics." In *AIDS: The Making of a Chronic Disease*. Berkeley: Univ. of California Press.

Decosas, Josef. 1991. Florence Conference Highlights: Social Epidemiology. *AIDS & Society* (July/August):7.

de la Vega, Ernesto. 1990. Considerations for Reaching the Latino Population with Sexuality and HIV/AIDS Information and Education. *SIECUS Report* (Sex Information and Education Council of the U.S.) 18 (February/March):1–22.

Demko, George J. 1990. AIDS in the USSR. *AIDS & Society* (April):4, 6.

Des Jarlais, Don C., and Samuel R. Friedman. 1989. AIDS and IV Drug Use. *Science* 245 (August 11):578.

Des Jarlais, Don C., et al. 1992. "The First City: HIV among Intravenous Drug Users in New York City." In *AIDS: The Making of a Chronic Disease*, edited by Elizabeth Fee and Daniel M. Fox. Berkeley: Univ. of California Press.

Desmond, Gerald. 1989. Economic Impact of AIDS in Developing Nations. *AIDS & Society* (October):5, 6.

Draper, William H. III. 1991. The Challenge of the HIV Epidemic. INDP infold in *AIDS & Society* (October/November):1.

Drucker, Ernest. 1991. "Communities at Risk: The Social Epidemiology of AIDS in New York City." In *AIDS and the Social Sciences*, edited by Richard Ulack and William F. Skinner. Lexington: Univ. Press of Kentucky.

Dubler, Nancy Neveloff, and Victor Seidel. 1991. "AIDS and the Prison System." In *A Disease of Society*, edited by Dorothy Nelkin et al. New York: Cambridge Univ. Press.

Earickson, Robert J. 1990. International Behavioral Responses to a Health Hazard: AIDS. *Social Science and Medicine:* 31(9):951–962.

Edgar, Harold, and David J. Rothman. 1991. "New Rules for New Drugs: The Challenge of AIDS to the Regulatory Process." In *A Disease of Society*, edited by Dorothy Nelkin et al. New York: Cambridge Univ. Press.

"Editorial: AIDS in Africa." 1988. In *The Heterosexual Transmission of AIDS in Africa*, edited by Dieter Koch-Weser and Hannelore

Vanderschmidt. Cambridge, Mass.: Abt Books.

Ehrhardt, Anke A. 1992. Trends in Sexual Behavior and the HIV Pandemic. *American Journal of Public Health* 82 (November):1459–1461.

Ergas, Yasmine. 1987. The Social Consequences of the AIDS Epidemic. Social Science Research Council, *Items* 41 (December):33–39.

Erlanger, Steven. 1991. A Plague Awaits. *New York Times Magazine* (July 14):24–26, 49, 53.

Farmer, Paul. 1990. "AIDS and Accusation: Haiti, Haitians, and the Geography of Blame." In *Culture and AIDS*, edited by Douglas A. Feldman. New York: Praeger.

Farmer, Paul. 1992. *AIDS and Accusation: Haiti and the Geography of Blame.* Berkeley: Univ. of California Press.

Fee, Elizabeth. 1988. "Sin versus Science: Venereal Disease in Twentieth-century Baltimore." In *AIDS: The Burdens of History*, edited by Elizabeth Fee and Daniel M. Fox. Berkeley: Univ. of California Press..

Fee, Elizabeth, and Daniel M. Fox, eds. 1988. *AIDS: The Burdens of History.* Berkeley: Univ. of California Press.

Fee, Elizabeth, and Daniel M. Fox, eds. 1992. *AIDS: The Making of a Chronic Disease.* Berkeley: Univ. of California Press.

Feldman, Douglas A., ed. 1990. *Culture and AIDS.* New York: Praeger.

Feldman, Douglas A. 1991. "The Sociocultural Impacts of AIDS in Central and East Africa." In *AIDS and the Social Sciences*, edited by Richard Ulack and William F. Skinner. Lexington: Univ. Press of Kentucky.

Fineberg, Harvey V. 1988a. Education to Prevent AIDS: Prospects and Obstacles. *Science* 239 (February 5):592–610.

Fineberg, Harvey V. 1988b. The Social Dimensions of AIDS. *Scientific American* 259 (October):128–134.

Fleming, Alan F. 1988. "Prevention of Transmission of HIV by Blood Transfusion in Developing Countries." In *The Global Impact of AIDS*, edited by Alan F. Fleming et al. New York: Alan R. Liss.

Fleming, Alan F., et al., eds. 1988. *The Global Impact of AIDS.* New York: Alan R. Liss.

Flowers, Nancy M. 1988. "The Spread of AIDS in Rural Brazil." In *AIDS 1988*, edited by Ruth Kulstad. Washington, D.C.: American Association for the Advancement of Science.

Focus: India. 1991. *AIDS & Society* (July/August):5.

Focus: Philippines. 1991. *AIDS & Society* (July/August):4.

Focus: Thailand. 1991. *AIDS & Society* (July/August):4.

Foege, William H. 1988. Plagues: Perceptions of Risk and Social Responses. *Social Research* 55 (3):331–342.

Foreman, Christopher H. Jr. 1993. What the AIDS Czar Can't Do. *New York Times* (July 14):A19.

Fortin, Alfred J. 1990. "AIDS, Development, and the Limitations of the African State." In *Action on AIDS*, edited by Barbara A. Misztal and David Moss. Westport, Conn.: Greenwood Press.

Fox, Daniel M. 1988a. "AIDS and the American Health Polity: The History and Prospects of a Crisis of Authority." In *AIDS: The Burdens of History*, edited by Elizabeth Fee and Daniel M. Fox. Berkeley: Univ. of California Press.

Fox, Daniel M. 1988b. "The Politics of Physicians' Responsibility in Epidemics: A Note on History." In *AIDS: The Burdens of History*, edited by Elizabeth Fee and Daniel M. Fox. Berkeley: Univ. of California Press.

Fox, Daniel M. 1992. "The Politics of HIV Infection: 1989–1990 as Years of Change." In *AIDS: The Making of a Chronic Disease*, edited by Elizabeth Fee and Daniel M. Fox. Berkeley: Univ. of California Press.

Fox, Daniel M., and Emily H. Thomas. 1990. "The Cost of AIDS: Exaggeration, Entitlement, and Economics." In *AIDS and the Health Care System*, edited by Lawrence O. Gostin. New Haven, Conn.: Yale Univ. Press.

Fox, Daniel M., et al. 1990. "The Power of Professionalism: Policies for AIDS in Britain, Sweden, and the United States." In *Living with AIDS*, edited by Stephen R. Graubard. Cambridge, Mass.: MIT Press.

Frankenburg, Ronald. 1988. "Social and Cultural Aspects of the Prevention of the Three Epidemics (HIV Infection, AIDS, and Counter-productive Societal Reaction to Them)." In *The Global Impact of AIDS*, edited by Alan F. Fleming et al. New York: Alan R. Liss.

Friedland, Gerald H. 1990. "Clinical Care in the AIDS Epidemic." In *Living with AIDS*, edited by Stephen R. Graubard. Cambridge, Mass.: MIT Press.

Friedman, Samuel R. 1991. "The Effects of AIDS on Intravenous Drug Users." In *A Disease of Society*, edited by Dorothy Nelkin et al. New York: Cambridge Univ. Press.

Friedman, Samuel R., et al. 1989. AIDS and the New Drug Injector. *Nature* 339 (June):333–334.

Fumento, Michael. 1989. The Incredible Shrinking AIDS Epidemic. *The American Spectator* (May):21–26.

Fumento, Michael. 1990. *The Myth of Heterosexual AIDS: How a Tragedy Has Been Distorted by the Media and Partisan Politics.* New York: Basic Books.

Gagnon, John H. 1990. "Disease and Desire." In *Living with AIDS,* edited by Stephen R. Graubard. Cambridge, Mass.: MIT Press.

Gallo, Robert C. 1991. *Virus Hunters: AIDS, Cancer, and the Human Retrovirus—A Story of Scientific Discovery.* New York: Basic Books.

Gallo, Robert C., and Luc Montagnier. 1988. The Authors Respond. *Scientific American* 260 (June):10–11.

Garrett, Laurie. 1992. "The Next Epidemic." In *AIDS in the World,* edited by Jonathan Mann et al., 825–839. Cambridge, Mass.: Harvard Univ. Press.

Gemson, Donald H., et al. 1991. Acquired Immunodeficiency Syndrome Prevention. *Archives of Internal Medicine* 151 (June):1102–1108.

Gerbert, Barbara, et al. 1989. Physicians and Acquired Immunodeficiency Virus: What Patients Think about Human Immunodeficiency Virus in Medical Practice. *Journal of the American Medical Association* 262 (October 16):1969–1972.

Gerbert, Barbara, et al. 1991a. The Impact of Who You Know and Where You Live on Opinions about AIDS and Health Care. *Social Science and Medicine* 32 (6):677–681.

Gerbert, Barbara, et al. 1991b. Primary Care Physicians and AIDS: Attitudinal and Structural Barriers to Care. *Journal of the American Medical Association* 266 (November 27):2837–2842.

Gil, Vicente E. 1990. Puerto Rico and the Caribbean. *AIDS & Society* (April):1, 8.

Goedert, James J. 1988. "The Natural History of HIV Infection." In *AIDS 1988,* edited by Ruth Kulstad. Washington, D.C.: American Association for the Advancement of Science.

Goldsmith, Marsha F. 1988. "AIDS around the World: Analyzing Complex Patterns." In *The Heterosexual Transmission of AIDS in Africa,* edited by Dieter Koch-Weser and Hannelore Vanderschmidt. Cambridge, Mass.: Abt Books.

Goldstein, Richard. 1991. "The Implicated and the Immune: Responses to AIDS in the Arts and Popular Culture." In *A Disease of Society,* edited by Dorothy Nelkin et al. New York: Cambridge Univ. Press.

Gostin, Lawrence O. 1986. The Future of Communicable Disease Control: Towards a New Concept in Public Health Law.

Milbank Quarterly 64 (Supplement 1):79–96.

Gostin, Lawrence O. 1987. "Traditional Public Health Strategies." In *AIDS and the Law*, edited by Harlon L. Dalton et al. New Haven, Conn.: Yale Univ. Press.

Gostin, Lawrence O. 1989. HIV-infected Physicians and the Practice of Seriously Invasive Procedures. *Hastings Center Report* (January–February):32–39.

Gostin, Lawrence O., ed. 1990a. *AIDS and the Health Care System.* New Haven, Conn.: Yale Univ. Press.

Gostin, Lawrence O. 1990b. "Preface: Hospitals, Health Care Professionals and Persons with AIDS." In *AIDS and the Health Care System*, edited by Lawrence O. Gostin. New Haven, Conn.: Yale Univ. Press.

Gostin, Lawrence O. 1992. "The AIDS Litigation Project: A National Review of Court and Human Rights Commission Decisions on Discrimination." In *AIDS: The Making of a Chronic Disease*, edited by Elizabeth Fee and Daniel M. Fox. Berkeley: Univ. of California Press.

Gostin, Lawrence, and William Curran. 1987. AIDS Screening, Confidentiality, and the Duty to Warn. *American Journal of Public Health* 77 (March):361365.

Gould, Peter. 1991. "Modeling the Geographic Spread of AIDS for Educational Intervention." In *AIDS and the Social Sciences*, edited by Richard Ulack and William F. Skinner. Lexington: Univ. Press of Kentucky.

Gould, Stephen Jay. 1991. "The Terrifying Normalcy of AIDS." In *The AIDS Reader*, edited by Nancy F. McKenzie. New York: Meridian. [First published in 1987.]

Graubard, Stephen R., ed. 1990. *Living with AIDS.* Cambridge, Mass.: MIT Press.

Grady, William R., et al. 1993. Condom Characteristics: The Perceptions and Preferences of Men in the United States. *Family Planning Perspectives* 25 (March/April):67–73.

Gray, Alec. 1989. "The AIDS Epidemic: A Prism Distorting Social and Legal Principles." In *The AIDS Epidemic*, edited by Padraig O'Malley. Boston: Beacon Press.

Green, Jesse, and Peter Arno. 1990. The "Medicaidization" of AIDS: Trends in the Financing of HIV-related Medical Care. *Journal of the American Medical Association* 264 (September 12):1261–1266.

Greenberg, Alan, et al. 1988. "The Association between Malaria, Blood Transfusions, and HIV Seropositivity in a Pediatric

Population in Kinshasa, Zaire." In *The Heterosexual Transmission of AIDS in Africa*, edited by Dieter Hoch-Weser and Hannelore Vanderschmidt. Cambridge, Mass.: Abt Books.

Griffiths, A. 1988. "Implications of the Medical and Scientific Aspects of HIV and AIDS for Economic Resourcing." In *The Global Impact of AIDS*, edited by Alan F. Fleming et al. New York: Alan R. Liss.

Grmek, Mirko D. 1990. *History of AIDS*. Princeton, N.J.; Princeton Univ. Press. [First published in 1989 as *Histoire du Sida*.]

Grodin, Michael A., et al. 1989. "Ethical Issues in AIDS Research." In *The AIDS Epidemic*, edited by Padraig O'Malley. Boston: Beacon Press.

Gruttola, Victor de, and William Ira Bennett. 1988. "Statistical Issues in Assessing the AIDS Epidemic." In *AIDS 1988*, edited by Ruth Kulstad. Washington, D.C.: American Association for the Advancement of Science.

Gruttola, Victor de, and William Ira Bennett. 1989. "AIDS: Prophecy and Present Reality." In *The AIDS Epidemic*, edited by Padraig O'Malley. Boston: Beacon Press.

Guydish, Joseph, et al. 1991. Evaluating Needle Exchange: Do Distributed Needles Come Back? *American Journal of Public Health* 81 (May):617–619.

Hale, John B. 1988 The Bishop's Blunder. *America* (February 13):158.

Hamburg, Margaret A., and Anthony S. Fauci. 1990. "AIDS: The Challenge to Biomedical Research." In *Living with AIDS*, edited by Stephen R. Graubard. Cambridge, Mass.: MIT Press.

Hammond, J. D., and Arnold F. Shapiro. 1986. AIDS and the Limits of Insurability. *Milbank Quarterly* 64 (Supplement 1):143–167.

Haq, Cynthia. 1988. "Management of AIDS Patients: Case Report from Uganda." In *AIDS in Africa*, edited by Norman N. Miller and Richard C. Rockwell. Lewiston, Me.: Edwin Mellen Press.

Hardy, Ann M., and Ann E. Biddlecom. 1991. "AIDS Knowledge and Attitudes of Black Americans: United States, 1990." A report of the National Center for Health Statistics. Hyattsville, Md.: The Center.

Haseltine, William A. 1990. "Prospects for the Medical Control of the AIDS Epidemic." In *Living with AIDS*, edited by Stephen R. Graubard. Cambridge, Mass.: MIT Press..

Haseltine, William A. 1992. Don't Bet on a Miracle. *New York Times* (November 15):IV19.

Haynes, Barton F. 1993. Scientific and Social Issues of Human

Immunodeficiency Virus Vaccine Development. *Science* 260 (May 28):1279–1286.

Heise, Lori. 1989. "Responding to AIDS." In *State of the World,* edited by Lester R. Brown et al. New York: Norton.

Hellinger, Fred J. 1991. Forecasting the Medical Care Costs of the HIV Epidemic: 1991–1992. *Inquiry* 28 (Fall):213–225.

Herman, Donald H. J. 1991. "AIDS and the Law." In *AIDS & Ethics,* edited by Frederic G. Reamer. New York: Columbia Univ. Press.

Herold, Edward S., and Carla van Kerkwijk. 1992. AIDS and Sex Tourism. *AIDS & Society* (October/November):1, 8.

Heyward, William L., and James W. Curran. 1988. The Epidemiology of AIDS in the U.S. *Scientific American* 259 (October):72–81.

Hinman, Alan R. 1991. Strategies to Prevent HIV Infection in the United States. *American Journal of Public Health* 81 (December):1557–1558.

HIV/AIDS Surveillance. A serial publication of the U.S. Public Health Service.

Hospedales, C. J., and S. Mahabir. 1988. "The Epidemiology of AIDS in the Caribbean and Action to Date." In *The Global Impact of AIDS,* edited by Alan F. Fleming et al. New York: Alan R. Liss.

Hospital Association of New York State. 1990. *The Impact of AIDS in New York State.* Executive Summary. Albany, N.Y.: The Association.

Hovitz, Jack A. de. 1988. "A Perspective on the Heterosexual Transmission of the Acquired Immunodeficiency Virus." In *The Heterosexual Transmission of AIDS in Africa,* edited by Dieter Koch-Weser and Hannelore Vanderschmidt. Cambridge, Mass.: Abt Books.

Hrdy, Daniel R. 1988. "Cultural Practices Contributing to the Transmission of Human Immunodeficiency Virus in Africa." In *The Heterosexual Transmission of AIDS in Africa,* edited by Dieter Koch-Weser and Hannelore Vanderschmidt. Cambridge, Mass.: Abt Books.

Huber, Joan, and Beth E. Schneider, eds. 1992. *The Social Context of AIDS.* Beverly Hills, Calif.: Sage Publications.

Hunt, Charles W. 1988. Africa and AIDS: Dependent Development, Sexism, and Racism. *Monthly Review* 39 (9):10–22.

Hunt, Charles W. 1989. Migrant Labor and Sexually Transmitted Disease: AIDS in Africa. *Journal of Health and Social Behavior* 30 (December):353–373.

Hunter, Nan D. 1990. *Epidemic of Fear: A Survey of AIDS Discrimination in the 1980's and Policy Recommendations for the 1990's*. New York: American Civil Liberties Union.

Ijsselmuiden, C., et al. 1993. AIDS in South Africa. *AIDS & Society* (January/February):1, 10–11.

Imperato, Pascal James. 1988. "The Epidemiology of the Acquired Immunodeficiency Syndrome in Africa." In *The Heterosexual Transmission of AIDS in Africa*, edited by Dieter Koch-Weser and Hannelore Vanderschmidt. Cambridge, Mass.: Abt Books.

Indian Blood Banks: An AIDS Depository? 1991. *AIDS & Society* (October/November):3.

Institute of Medicine, National Academy of Sciences. 1986a. *Confronting AIDS: Directions for Public Health, Health Care, and Research*. Washington, D.C.: National Academy Press.

Institute of Medicine, National Academy of Sciences. 1986b. *Mobilizing against AIDS: The Unfinished Story of a Virus*. Written by Eve K. Nichols. Cambridge, Mass.: Harvard Univ. Press.

Institute of Medicine, National Academy of Sciences. 1991. "Behavioral Interventions for the Prevention of Sexual Transmission of HIV." A report of the International Forum for AIDS Research. Infold in *AIDS & Society* (May).

Jasny, Barbara R. 1993. AIDS 1993: The Unanswered Questions. *Science* 260 (May 28):1219.

Johnston, Margaret I., and Daniel F. Hoth. 1993. Present Status and Future Prospects for HIV Therapies. *Science* 260 (May 28):1286–1293.

Jonsen, Albert R. 1990. "The Duty to Treat Patients with AIDS and HIV Infection." In *AIDS and the Health Care System*, edited by Lawrence O. Gostin. New Haven, Conn.: Yale Univ. Press.

Jonsen, Albert R., and Jeff Stryker, eds. 1993. *The Social Impact of AIDS in the United States*. Washington, D.C.: National Academy Press.

Kass, Frederic C. 1987. "Schoolchildren with AIDS." In *AIDS and the Law*, edited by Harlon L. Dalton et al. New Haven, Conn.: Yale Univ. Press.

Kateb, George. 1988. Moral Dilemmas—An Introduction. *Social Research* 55 (3): 455-460.

Keniston, Kenneth. 1990. "Introduction to the Issue." In *Living with AIDS*, edited by Stephen R. Graubard. Cambridge, Mass.: MIT Press.

Khan, M. E., et al. 1991. India's Epidemic. *AIDS & Society* (July/August):5.

Killip, Thomas. 1989. "Hospitals in New York City: A System under Stress." In *Public and Professional Attitudes toward AIDS Patients*, edited by David E. Rogers and Eli Ginzburg. Boulder, Colo.: Westview Press.

Kinsella, James. 1990. *Covering the Plague: AIDS and the American Media*. New Brunswick, N.J.: Rutgers Univ. Press.

Kirby, Michael. 1990. "AIDS and the Law." In *Living with AIDS*, edited by Stephen R. Graubard. Cambridge, Mass.: MIT Press.

Kirp, David L., and Ronald Bayer, eds. 1992. *AIDS in the Industrialized Democracies: Passions, Politics, and Policy*. New Brunswick, N.J.: Rutgers Univ. Press.

Klepinger, Daniel H. et al. 1993. Perceptions of AIDS Risk and Severity and Their Association with Risk-related Behavior among U.S. Men. *Family Planning Perspectives* 25(March/April):74–82.

Kobasa, Suzanne C. Ouellette. 1991. "AIDS and Voluntary Associations." In *A Disease of Society*, edited by Dorothy Nelkin et al. New York: Cambridge Univ. Press.

Koch-Weser, Dieter. 1988. "Introduction." In *The Heterosexual Transmission of AIDS in Africa*, edited by Dieter Koch-Weser and Hannelore Vanderschmidt. Cambridge, Mass.: Abt Books.

Koch-Weser, Dieter, and Hannelore Vanderschmidt, eds. 1988. *The Heterosexual Transmission of AIDS in Africa*. Cambridge, Mass.: Abt Books.

Koop, C. Everett. 1986. *Report on AIDS*. Washington, D.C.: Office of the Surgeon General.

Krause, Richard M. 1992. The Origin of Plagues: Old and New. *Science* 257 (August 21):1073–1077.

Krisber, Paul, and Harry Blaney. 1987. AIDS International: Disease Is Altering the Nation's Foreign Policy. *The Bergen (N.J.) Record.* (October 16). [Reprinted from the *Washington Post.*]

Kuller, Lewis H., and Lawrence A. Kingsley. 1986. The Epidemic of AIDS: A Failure of Public Health Policy. *Milbank Quarterly* 64 (Supplement 1):56-78.

Kulstad, Ruth, ed. 1988. *AIDS 1988: AAAS Symposia Papers*. Washington, D.C.: American Association for the Advancement of Science.

Lamb, George A., and Linette G. Liebling. 1989. "The Role of Education in AIDS Prevention." In *The AIDS Epidemic*, edited by Padraig O'Malley. Boston: Beacon Press.

Lambda Legal Defense and Education Fund. 1987. *Living with AIDS: A Layperson's Guide to the Legal Problems of People with AIDS.*

New York: The Fund.

Lederberg, Joshua. 1988. Pandemic as a Natural Evolutionary Phenomenon. *Social Research* 55 (3):343-360.

Lee, Deborah A., and Kevin Fong. 1990. HIV/AIDS and the Asian and Pacific Islander Community. *SIECUS Report* (Sex Information and Education Council of the U.S.) 18 (February/March):16-22.

Leonard, Arthur S. 1987. "AIDS in the Workplace." In *AIDS and the Law*, edited by Harlon L. Dalton et al. New Haven, Conn.: Yale Univ. Press.

Levine, Carol. 1990a. "In and Out of the Hospital." In *AIDS and the Health Care System*, edited by Lawrence O. Gostin. New Haven, Conn.: Yale Univ. Press.

Levine, Carol. 1990b. Women and HIV/AIDS Research: The Barriers to Equity. *Evaluation Review* 14 (October):447–463.

Levine, Carol. 1991. "AIDS and Changing Concepts of Family." In *A Disease of Society*, edited by Dorothy Nelkin et al. New York: Cambridge Univ. Press.

Levine, Carol, and Ronald Bayer. 1989. The Ethics of Screening for Early Intervention in HIV Disease. *American Journal of Public Health* 79 (December):1661–1667.

Levy, Judith A., and Gary L. Albrecht. 1989. "A Review of Research on Sexual and AIDS-related Attitudes and Behaviors." In *AIDS in an Aging Society*, edited by Matilda White Riley et al. New York: Springer.

Lloyd, Robin. 1988. "Looking Back and Forward: Hospital Responses." In *The Social Impact of AIDS in the U.S.*, edited by Richard A. Berk. Cambridge, Mass.: Abt Books.

A Lost Generation. 1993. *Newsweek* (January 18):16–20.

Ludmerer, Kenneth M. 1989. "Patients Beyond the Pale: A Historical View." In *Public and Professional Attitudes toward AIDS Patients*, edited by David E. Rogers and Eli Ginzburg. Boulder, Colo.: Westview Press.

Lyon, Jeff. 1992. "Keeping Score: A University of Chicago Research Team Is Exploring Sexual America." *Chicago Tribune Magazine* (November 29):14-16, 28–34.

McArthur, Justin C. 1992. "Dementia and Other Neurological Manifestations of HIV/AIDS." In *AIDS in the World*, edited by Jonathan Mann et al., 678-683. Cambridge, Mass.: Harvard Univ. Press.

McDermott, Jim. 1991. Asia—The Smoldering Volcano. *AIDS & Society* (July/August):1, 4.

McKenzie, Nancy F., ed. 1991. *The AIDS Reader: Social, Political, and Economic Issues*. New York: Meridian.

McKinlay, John B., et al. 1989. "On the Relevance of Social Science Concepts and Perspectives." In *AIDS in an Aging Society*, edited by Matilda White Riley et al. New York: Springer.

McLaughlin, Loretta. 1989. "AIDS: An Overview." In *The AIDS Epidemic*, edited by Padraig O'Malley. Boston: Beacon Press.

McNeill, William H. 1976. *Plagues and People*. Garden City, N.Y.: Doubleday.

Maddox, George L., and G. David Maddox. 1989. "The Complementarity of Psychosocial and Biomedical Research on AIDS." In *AIDS in an Aging Society*, edited by Matilda White Riley et al. New York: Springer.

Mandelker, Daniel R. 1987. "Housing Issues." In *AIDS and the Law*, edited by Harlon L. Dalton et al. New Haven, Conn.: Yale Univ. Press.

Mann, Jonathan. 1988a. Interview: Jonathan Mann. *AIDS Patient Care* (June):16–19.

Mann, Jonathan. 1988b. "The Global Picture of AIDS." Unpublished paper delivered at the Fourth International Conference on AIDS, Stockholm. June 12–16.

Mann, Jonathan. 1988c. "Worldwide Epidemiology of AIDS." In *The Global Impact of AIDS*, edited by Alan F. Fleming et al. New York: Alan R. Liss.

Mann, Jonathan. 1989a. "Global AIDS into the 1990's." Unpublished paper delivered at the Fifth International Conference on AIDS, Montreal, June 4–9.

Mann, Jonathan. 1989b. Global AIDS into the 1990s. *World Health*: (October):6–7.

Mann, Jonathan. 1989c. "Global AIDS: Epidemic at a Crossroads." Press release. Geneva: World Health Organization. November.

Mann, Jonathan. 1991a. AIDS and the Next Pandemic. *Scientific American* (March):126.

Mann, Jonathan. 1991b. Where Are We Now? AIDS. *Health Policy and Planning*: 6 (2):191–193.

Mann, Jonathan et al. 1988. "The International Epidemiology of AIDS." *Scientific American* (October):82–89.

Mann, Jonathan, et al., eds. 1992. *AIDS in the World*. Cambridge, Mass.: Harvard Univ. Press.

Marin, Gerardo. 1989. AIDS Prevention among Hispanics: Needs, Risk Behaviors, and Cultural Values. *Public Health Reports* (September/October):411–415.

Marx, Jean L. 1989. Circumcision May Protect against the AIDS Virus. *Science* 245 (August 4):470–471.

May, Robert M., et al. 1990. "The Epidemiology and Transmission Dynamics of HIV-AIDS." In *Living with AIDS*, edited by Stephen R. Graubard. Cambridge, Mass.: MIT Press.

Mayer, Kenneth H. 1988. "Public Policy Implications of the Natural History of HIV Infection." In *AIDS 1988*, edited by Ruth Kulstad. Washington, D.C.: American Association for the Advancement of Science.

Mays, Vickie M., and Susan D. Cochran. 1988. Issues in the Perception of AIDS Risk and Risk Reduction Activities by Black and Hispanic/Latina Women. *American Psychologist* 43 (November):949–957.

Mazur, Bridget. 1991. Latin America and the Caribbean: Puzzling New Patterns of HIV Transmission. *AIDS & Society* (April/May):1, 6–7.

Mazur, Bridget. 1992. "The Cuba Experience: Is AIDS Eradication Possible?" *AIDS & Society* (January/February):1, 8–9, 11.

Merson, Michael H. 1993. Slowing the Spread of AIDS: Agenda for the 1990s. *Science* 260 (May 28):1266-1268.

Michaels, David, and Carol Levine. 1992. Estimates of the Number of Motherless Youth Orphaned by AIDS in the United States. *Journal of the American Medical Association* 268 (December 23/30):3456–3461.

Miike, Lawrence, et al. 1991. *AIDS in the Health Care Workplace.* Washington, D.C.: Office of Technology Assessment.

Miller, Heather G., et al., eds. 1990. *AIDS: The Second Decade.* Washington, D.C.: National Academy Press.

Miller, Norman N. 1992. Jonathan's Report Card. *AIDS & Society* (July/August):3.

Miller, Norman N., and Manuel Carballo. 1989. AIDS: A Disease of Development? *AIDS & Society* (October):1, 21.

Miller, Norman H., and Richard C. Rockwell, eds. 1988a. *AIDS in Africa: Emerging Issues and Social Implications.* Lewiston, Me.: Edwin Mellen Press.

Miller, Norman H., and Richard C. Rockwell. 1988b. "Introduction." In *AIDS in Africa*, edited by Norman N. Miller and Richard C. Rockwell. Lewiston, Me.: Edwin Mellen Press.

Mirante, Edith T. 1992. Burma's AIDS Epidemic. *AIDS & Society* (July/August):1, 6–7.

Misztal, Barbara, and David Moss, eds. 1990. *Action on AIDS: National Policies in Comparative Perspective.* Westport, Conn.:

Greenwood Press.

Morbidity and Mortality Weekly Report (MMWR). A serial publication of the U.S. Public Health Service.

Moran, John S., et al. 1989. The Impact of Sexually Transmitted Diseases on Minority Populations. *Public Health Reports* (November/December):560–565.

Morse, Stephen S. 1992. "AIDS and Beyond: Defining the Rules for Viral Traffic." In *AIDS: The Making of a Chronic Disease,* edited by Elizabeth Fee and Daniel M. Fox. Berkeley: Univ. of California Press.

Morton, Oliver, et al. 1992. "Achievements in Research." In *AIDS in the World,* edited by Jonathan Mann et al., 229—275. Cambridge, Mass.: Harvard Univ. Press.

Muhondwa, E.P.Y. 1991. Youth, Disbelief, and Fatalism in Tanzania. *AIDS & Society* (April/May):10–11.

Mulera, Muniini. 1989. Letter to the Editors. *Scientific American* 26 (June):10.

Murphy, Julien S. 1988. "Women with AIDS: Sexual Ethics of an Epidemic." In *AIDS: Principles, Practices, & Politics,* edited by Inge B. Corless and Mary Pittman-Lindeman. Washington, D.C.: Hemisphere Publishing Corp.

Murphy, Timothy F. 1991. No Time for an AIDS Backlash. *Hastings Center Report* (March–April):7–11.

Murray, Thomas H. 1991. "The Poisoned Gift: AIDS and Blood." In *A Disease of Society,* edited by Dorothy Nelkin et al. New York: Cambridge Univ. Press.

Musto, David F. 1988. "Quarantine and the Problem of AIDS." In *AIDS: The Burdens of History,* edited by Elizabeth Fee and Daniel M. Fox. Berkeley: Univ. of California Press.

Mutambirwo, Jane. 1992. "Aspects of Sexual Behavior in Local Cultures and the Transmission of Sexually Transmitted Diseases (STDs) Including AIDS." Unpublished paper delivered to the Anthropology Group Session on Culture, Sexual Behavior, and AIDS at the Eighth International Conference on AIDS, Amsterdam, July 24–26, 1992.

National Commission on AIDS. 1989. "Failure of U.S. Health Care System to Deal with HIV Epidemic." Interim Report No. 1, December. Washington, D.C.: The Commission.

National Commission on AIDS. 1990a. "Leadership, Legislation, and Regulation." Interim Report No. 2, April. Washington, D.C.: The Commission.

National Commission on AIDS. 1990b. "Research, the Work Force, and the HIV Epidemic in Rural America." Interim Report No. 3, August. Washington, D.C.: The Commission.

National Commission on AIDS. 1991a. "HIV Disease in Correctional Facilities." Interim Report No. 4, March. Washington, D.C.: The Commission.

National Commission on AIDS. 1991b. "The Twin Epidemics of Substance Use and HIV." Interim Report No. 5, July. Washington, D.C.: The Commission.

National Commission on AIDS. 1991c. *America Living with AIDS: Transforming Anger, Fear, and Indifference into Action.* Washington, D.C.: The Commission.

National Commission on AIDS. 1992a. "Preventing HIV Transmission in Health Care Settings." Washington, D.C.: The Commission.

National Commission on AIDS. 1992b *The Challenge of HIV/AIDS in Communities of Color.* January. Washington, D.C.: The Commission.

National Commisssion on AIDS. 1993. *AIDS: An Expanding Tragedy.* Final Report, June. Includes Cumulative Recommendations and indexed Guide to Commission Reports. Washington, D.C. The Commission.

Nelkin, Dorothy, and Sander L. Gilman. 1988. Placing Blame for Devastating Disease. *Social Research* 55 (3):361–378.

Nelkin, Dorothy, and Stephen Hilgartner. 1986. Disputed Dimensions of Risk: A Public School Controversy over AIDS. *Milbank Quarterly* 64 (Supplement 1):118–142.

Nelkin, Dorothy, et al., eds. 1991. *A Disease of Society: Cultural and Institutional Responses to AIDS.* Cambridge Univ. Press.

Nelson, Nici. 1988. "Selling Her Kiosk: Kikuyo Notions of Sexuality and Sex for Sale in Mathera Valley, Kenya." In *The Cultural Construction of Sexuality,* edited by Pat Caplan. London: Tavistock Publications.

Ness, Roberta, et al. 1989. Likelihood of Contact with AIDS Patients as a Factor in Medical Students' Residency Selections. *Academic Medicine* 64 (October):588–594.

Ness, Roberta, et al. 1991. House Staff Recruitment to Municipal and Voluntary New York City Residency Programs during the AIDS Epidemic. *Journal of the American Medical Association* 266 (November 27):2843–2846.

Newsbriefs: United States. 1992. *AIDS & Society* (April/May):3.

Nkowane, Benjamin M. 1988. "The Impact of Human Immunodeficiency Virus Infection and AIDS on a Primary Industry:

Mining (A Case Study of Zambia)." In *The Global Impact of AIDS*, edited by Alan F. Fleming et al. New York: Alan R. Liss.

NORC [National Opinion Research Center, University of Chicago]. 1987. Unpublished proposal for a nationwide survey of sexual behavior. Chicago: NORC.

NORC [National Opinion Research Center, University of Chicago]. 1992. Sex Survey Conducted. *The NORC Reporter:* 6 (Fall):8.

Nordberg, Olivia Schieffelin. 1933. What Do the Men Say? *Family Planning Perspectives* 25 (March/April):Inside cover.

Nyonyintono, Namuli. 1992. Report from Uganda: The Impact of HIV/AIDS on the Lives of Children. *AIDS & Society* (January/February):6–7.

O'Malley, Padraig, ed. 1989. *The AIDS Epidemic: Private Rights and the Public Interest.* Boston: Beacon Press.

O'Neill, Catherine. 1987. "Intravenous Drug Users." In *AIDS and the Law,* edited by Harlon L. Dalton et al. New Haven, Conn.: Yale Univ. Press.

Oppenheimer, Gerald M. 1988. "In the Eye of the Storm: The Epidemiological Construction of AIDS." In *AIDS: The Burdens of History,* edited by Elizabeth Fee and Daniel M. Fox. Berkeley: Univ. of California Press.

Oppenheimer, Gerald M. 1992. "Causes, Cases, and Cohorts: The Role of Epidemiology in the Historical Construction of AIDS." In *AIDS: The Burdens of History,* edited by Elizabeth Fee and Daniel M. Fox. Berkeley: Univ. of California Press.

Oppenheimer, Gerald M., and Robert A. Padgug. 1991. "AIDS and the Crisis of Health Insurance." In *AIDS & Ethics,* edited by Frederic G. Reamer. New York: Columbia Univ. Press.

Osborn, June E. 1990. "Public Health and the Politics of AIDS Prevention." In *Living with AIDS,* edited by Stephen R. Graubard. Cambridge, Mass.: MIT Press.

Ostrow, David G. 1990. "AIDS Prevention through Effective Education." In *Living with AIDS,* edited by Stephen R. Graubard. Cambridge, Mass: MIT Press.

PAACNOTES. 1991. "Do Physicians and Dentists Have an Obligation to Disclose Their HIV Status before Invasive Surgery?" Chicago: Physicians Association for AIDS Care.

Packard, Randall M., and Paul Epstein. 1992. "Medical Research on AIDS in Africa: A Historical Perspective." In *AIDS: The Making of a Chronic Disease,* edited by Elizabeth Fee and Daniel M. Fox. Berkeley: Univ. of California Press.

Padgug, Robert A., and Gerald M. Oppenheimer. 1992. "Riding the

Tiger: AIDS and the Gay Community." In *AIDS: The Making of a Chronic Disease*, edited by Elizabeth Fee and Daniel M. Fox. Berkeley: Univ. of California Press.

Paintal, A. S. 1989. Interview: It Is Women Who Are the Lousy Lot. *Sunday* (Calcutta):16 (February 26–March 4).

Pakistani Enigma: AIDS Education. 1992. *AIDS & Society* (January/February):3.

Panem, Sandra. 1988. *The AIDS Bureaucracy: Why Society Failed to Meet the AIDS Crisis and How We Might Improve Our Response.* Cambridge, Mass.: Harvard Univ. Press.

Panos Dossier. 1989. *AIDS and the Third World.* Published in association with the Norwegian Red Cross by the Panos Institute. Philadelphia: New Society Publishers.

Parker, Richard G. 1988. "Sexual Culture and AIDS Education in Urban Brazil." In *AIDS: 1988*, edited by Ruth Kulstad. Washington, D.C.: American Association for the Advancement of Science.

Parker, Richard G. 1990. "Responding to AIDS in Brazil." In *Action on AIDS*, edited by Barbara A. Misztal and David Moss. Westport, Conn.: Greenwood Press.

Parker, Richard G. 1991. *Bodies, Pleasures, and Passions: Sexual Culture in Contemporary Brazil.* Boston: Beacon Press.

Peck, Jonathan, and Clement Bezold. 1992. Health Care and AIDS. American Academy of Political and Social Science, *Annals* 522 (July):130–139.

Pérez-Stable, Eliseo J. 1991. Cuba's Response to the HIV Epidemic. *American Journal of Public Health* 81 (May): 563-566.

Perrow, Charles, and Mauro F. Guillén. 1990. *The AIDS Disaster: The Failure of Organizations in New York and the Nation.* New Haven, Conn.: Yale Univ. Press.

Pescosolido, Bernice A., et al., eds. 1991. *The Sociology of AIDS: Six Lectures and Materials for Instructors and Students.* Washington, D.C.: American Sociological Association Teaching Resources Center.

Peterson, J. L., et al. 1992. High Risk Sexual Behavior and Condom Use among Gay and Bisexual African-American Men. *American Journal of Public Health* 82 (November):1490–1494.

Pierce, Christine, and Donald VanDeVeer, eds. 1988. *AIDS: Ethics and Public Policy.* Belmont, Calif.: Wadsworth Publishing Co.

Pietrow, Phyllis L., et al. 1992. "AIDS and Mass Persuassion." In *AIDS in the World*, edited by Jonathan Mann et al., 733–747. Cambridge, Mass.: Harvard Univ. Press.

Piot, Peter, et al. 1988a. AIDS: An International Perspective. *Science* 239 (February 5):573–579.

Piot, Peter, et al. 1988b. "Heterosexual Transmission of HIV." In *The Heterosexual Transmission of AIDS in Africa*, edited by Dieter Koch-Weser and Hannelore Vanderschmidt. Cambridge, Mass.: Abt Books.

Poirier, Richard. 1988. AIDS and Traditions of Homophobia. *Social Research* 55 (3):461–476.

Pollak, Michael. 1990. "AIDS Policy in France: Biomedical Leadership and Preventive Impotence." In *Action on AIDS*, edited by Barbara A. Misztal and David Moss. Westport, Conn.: Greenwood Press.

Porter, Dorothy, and Roy Porter. 1988. "The Enforcement of Health: The British Debate." In *AIDS: The Burdens of History*, edited by Elizabeth Fee and Daniel M. Fox. Berkeley: Univ. of California Press.

Porter, Veneita. 1989. "Minorities and HIV Infection." In *The AIDS Epidemic*, edited by Padraig O'Malley. Boston: Beacon Press.

Presidential Commission on the Human Immunodeficiency Virus Epidemic. 1988. *Report*. Submitted to the President of the United States, June 24, 1988. Washington, D.C.: U.S. Government Printing Office. [Known as the Watkins Report.]

Prewitt, Kenneth. 1988. "Foreword." In *AIDS in Africa*, edited by Norman N. Miller and Richard C. Rockwell. Lewiston, Me.: Edwin Mellen Press.

Quetel, Claude. 1990. *History of Syphilis*. New York: Oxford Univ. Press.

Quinn, Thomas C., et al. 1986. AIDS in Africa: An Epidemiological Paradigm. *Science* 234 (November 21):955–963.

Quinton, Anthony. 1988. Plagues and Morality. *Social Research* 55 (3):477-490.

Reamer, Frederic G., ed. 1991. *AIDS & Ethics*. New York: Columbia Univ. Press.

Redfield, Robert R., and Donald S. Burke. 1988. HIV Infection: The Clinical Picture. *Scientific American* 259 (October):90–98.

Richards, David A. J. 1988. Human Rights, Public Health, and the Idea of Moral Plague. *Social Research* 55 (3):491–509.

Riley, Matilda White. 1989. "AIDS and Older People: The Overlooked Segment of the Population." In *AIDS in an Aging Society*, edited by Matilda White Riley et al. New York: Springer.

Riley, Matilda White et al., eds. 1989. *AIDS in an Aging Society: What We Need to Know*. New York: Springer.

Risse, Guenter B. 1988. "Epidemics and History: Ecological Perspectives and Social Responses." In *AIDS: The Burdens of History,* edited by Elizabeth Fee and Daniel M. Fox. Berkeley: Univ. of California Press.

Rivera, Rhonda R. 1987. "The Military." In *AIDS and the Law,* edited by Harlon L. Dalton et al. New Haven, Conn.: Yale Univ. Press.

Rizzo, John A., et al. 1990. Physician Contact with and Attitudes toward HIV-seropositive Patients: Results from a National Survey. *Medical Care* 28 (March):251–259.

Rockwell, Richard C. 1988. Social Impacts of the HIV Epidemic. *AIDS* 2 (Supplement 1):5223–5227.

Rockwell, Richard C. 1989. "The Socioeconomic Impacts of AIDS: Many Questions, Few Answers." Unpublished paper. New York: Social Science Research Council.

Rogers, David E. 1992. Report Card on Our National Response to the AIDS Epidemic—Some A's, Too Many D's. *American Journal of Public Health* 82 (April):522–524.

Rogers, David E., and Eli Ginzburg, eds. 1989. *Public and Professional Attitudes toward AIDS Patients: A National Dilemma.* Boulder, Colo.: Westview Press.

Rogers, Everett M., et al. 1991. AIDS in the 1990's: The Agenda-setting Process for a Public Issue. *Journalism Monographs* 126 (April):1–47.

Ron, Aron, and David E. Rogers. 1990. "AIDS in the United States: Patient Care and Politics." In *Living with AIDS,* edited by Stephen R. Graubard. Cambridge, Mass.: MIT Press.

Rosenberg, Charles E. 1988a. The Definition and Control of Disease—An Introduction. *Social Research* 55 (3):327–330.

Rosenberg, Charles E. 1988b. "Disease and Social Order in America: Perceptions and Expectations." In *AIDS: The Burdens of History,* edited by Elizabeth Fee and Daniel M. Fox. Berkeley: Univ. of California Press.

Rosenberg, Charles E. 1990. "What Is an Epidemic? AIDS in Historical Perspective." In *Living with AIDS,* edited by Stephen R. Graubard. Cambridge, Mass.: MIT Press.

Rosenkrantz, Barbara Gutman. 1988. Case Histories—An Introduction. *Social Research* 55 (3):397–400.

Rothman, David J., and Harold Edgar. 1992. "Scientific Rigor and Medical Realities: Placebo Trials in Cancer and AIDS Research." In *AIDS: The Making of a Chronic Disease,* edited by Elizabeth Fee and Daniel M. Fox. Berkeley: Univ. of California Press.

Rothstein, Mark A. 1987. "Screening Workers for AIDS." In *AIDS and the Law*, edited by Harlon L. Dalton et al. New Haven, Conn.: Yale Univ. Press.

Rowell, Ronald M. 1990. Native Americans, Stereotypes, and HIV/AIDS: Our Continuing Struggle for Survival. *SIECUS Report* (Sex Information and Education Council of the U.S.) 18 (February/March):9–15.

Rutayuga, John. 1992a. To the Editor. *AIDS & Society* (April/May):2.

Rutayuga, John. 1992b. Traditional Medicine and AIDS. *AIDS & Society* (April/May):5.

Sabatier, Renée, et al. 1988. *Blaming Others: Prejudice, Race and Worldwide AIDS*. Published in association with the Norwegian Red Cross by the Panos Institute. Santa Cruz, Calif.: New Society West.

Sapolsky, Harvey M. 1990. "AIDS, Blood Banking, and the Bonds of Community." In *Living with AIDS*, edited by Stephen R. Graubard. Cambridge, Mass.: MIT Press.

Sapolsky, Harvey M., and Stephen L. Boswell. 1992. "The History of Transfusion AIDS: Practice and Policy Alternatives." In *AIDS: The Making of a Chronic Disease*, edited by Elizabeth Fee and Daniel M. Fox. Berkeley: Univ. of California Press.

Schatz, Benjamin. 1991. "'May God and the Community Help Us All': Results of a Survey of HIV-positive and 'High Risk' Untested Health Care Workers." San Francisco: Medical Expertise Retention Program.

Scheinman, David, et al. 1992. Treating AIDS with Traditional Medicine. *AIDS & Society* (April/May):5.

Scherzer, Mark. 1987. "Insurance." In *AIDS and the Law*, edited by Harlon L. Dalton et al. New Haven, Conn.: Yale Univ. Press.

Schoepf, Brooke Grundfest, et al. 1988a. "AIDS, Women, and Society in Central Africa." In *AIDS 1988*, edited by Ruth Kulstad. Washington, D.C.: American Association for the Advancement of Science.

Schoepf, Brooke Grundfest, et al. 1988b. "AIDS and Society in Central Africa: A View from Zaire." In *AIDS in Africa*, edited by Norman N. Miller and Richard C. Rockwell. Lewiston, Me.: Edwin Mellen Press.

Schoepf, Brooke Grundfest, et al. 1991. "Gender, Power, and Risk of AIDS in Zaire." In *Women and Health in Africa*, edited by Meredeth Turshen. Trenton, N.J.: Africa World Press.

Schwarz, M. Roy. 1989. "Physicians' Attitudes Toward AIDS." In *Public and Professional Attitudes toward AIDS Patients*, edited by David E. Rogers and Eli Ginzburg. Boulder, Colo.: Westview Press.

Scitovsky, Anne A. 1988. "Estimates of the Direct and Indirect Costs of AIDS in the United States." In *The Global Impact of AIDS,* edited by Alan F. Fleming et al. New York: Alan R. Liss.

Second Public Health Service AIDS Prevention and Control Conference. 1988. Report. *Public Health Reports* 103 (Supplement 1):1–109.

Selik, Richard M., et al. 1988. "Epidemiology of AIDS and HIV Infection in the United States." In *The Global Impact of AIDS,* edited by Alan F. Fleming et al. New York: Alan R. Liss.

Shapiro, Martin F., et al. 1992. Residents' Experiences in, and Attitudes Toward, the Care of Persons with AIDS in Canada, France, and the United States. *Journal of the American Medical Association* 264 (July 22–29):510–515.

Shilts, Randy. 1987. *And the Band Played On: Politics, People, and the AIDS Epidemic.* New York: St. Martin's Press.

Siegel, Karolyn, and William C. Gibson. 1988. Barriers to Modification of Sexual Behavior among Heterosexuals at Risk for Acquired Immunodeficiency Syndrome. *New York State Journal of Medicine* 88 (February):66–70.

Sills, David L. [1957] 1980. *The Volunteers: Means and Ends in a National Organization.* New York: Arno Press.

Simpson, Michael A. 1988. "The Malignant Metaphor: A Political Thanatology of AIDS." In *AIDS: Principles, Practices, & Politics,* edited by Inge B. Corless and Mary Pittman-Lindeman. Washington, D.C.: Hemisphere Publishing Corp.

Singer, Eleanor, et al. 1991. Changes in Public Opinion about AIDS. *Public Opinion Quarterly* 55:161–179.

Singer, Eleanor, et al. 1993. "Public Opinion about AIDS Before and After the U. S. Government's Public Information Campaign." *Public Opinion Quarterly.* In press.

Sisk, Jane E., et al. 1988. *The Effectiveness of AIDS Education.* Washington, D.C.: Office of Technology Assessment.

Slack, Paul. 1988. Responses to Plague in Early Modern Europe: The Implications of Public Health. *Social Research* 55 (3):433–453.

Slutsker, Laurence, et al. 1992. "The Shape of the Pandemic: Trends in the United States and Europe." In *AIDS in the World,* edited by Jonathan Mann et al., 605–616. Cambridge, Mass.: Harvard Univ. Press.

Smallman-Raynor, M.R., and A.D. Cliff. 1991. Civil War and the

Spread of AIDS in Central Africa. *Epidemiology of Infections* 107:69–80.

Sontag, Susan. 1978. *Illness as Metaphor.* New York: Vintage Press.

Sontag, Susan. 1988. *AIDS and Its Metaphors.* New York: Farrar, Strauss and Giroux.

Stall, Ron, et al. 1992. "Maintenance of HIV Risk Reduction among Gay-identified Men." In *AIDS in the World,* edited by Jonathan Mann et al., 653-657. Cambridge, Mass.: Harvard Univ. Press.

Stoddard, Thomas B., and Walter Rieman. 1991. "AIDS and the Rights of the Individual: Toward a More Sophisticated Understanding of Discrimination." In *A Disease of Society,* edited by Dorothy Nelkin et al. New York: Cambridge Univ. Press.

Strauss, Anselm L., et al. 1991. AIDS and Health Care Deficiencies. *Society* (July/August):63–73.

Street, John, and Albert Weale. 1992. "Britain: Policy-making in a Hermetically Sealed System." In *AIDS in the Industrialized Democracies,* edited by David L. Kirp and Ronald Bayer. New Brunswick, N.J.: Rutgers Univ. Press.

Swenson, Robert M. 1988. Plagues, History, and AIDS. *American Scholar* 57 (Spring):183–200.

Tanfer, Koray, et al. 1993. Condom Use among U.S. Men. *Family Planning Perspectives* 25(March/April):61–66.

Tarantola, D. 1988. "Global Strategy for the Prevention and Control of AIDS." In *The Global Impact of AIDS,* edited by Alan F. Fleming et al. New York: Alan R. Liss.

Tauer, Carol A. 1988. "AIDS and Human Rights: An Intercontinental Perspective." In *AIDS: Ethics and Public Policy,* edited by Christine Pierce and Donald VanDeVeer. Belmont, Calif.: Wadsworth Publishing Co.

Thier, Samuel O. 1988. "Foreword." In *The AIDS Bureaucracy,* by Sandra Panem. Cambridge, Mass.: Harvard Univ. Press.

Thomas, Lewis. 1988. Science and Health—Possibilities, Probabilities, and Limitations. *Social Research* 55 (3):379–396.

Thomas, Lewis. 1989. "AIDS: A Long View." In *Public and Professional Attitudes toward AIDS Patients,* edited by David E. Rogers and Eli Ginzburg. Boulder, Colo.: Westview Press.

Tomasevski, Katarina. 1992. "AIDS and Human Rights." In *AIDS in the World,* edited by Jonathan Mann et al., 538–573. Cambridge, Mass.: Harvard Univ. Press.

Torrey, Barbara Boyle, et al. 1988. " Epidemiology of HIV and AIDS in Africa: Emerging Issues and Social Implications." In *AIDS in Africa,* edited by Norman N. Miller and Richard C. Rockwell. Lewiston, Me.: Edwin Mellen Press.

Treichler, Paula A. 1988. "AIDS, Gender, and Biomedical Discourse: Current Contests for Meaning" In *AIDS: The Burdens of History,* edited by Elizabeth Fee and Daniel M. Fox. Berkeley: Univ. of California Press.

Treichler, Paula A. 1992. "AIDS and HIV Infection in the Third World: A First World Chronicle." In *AIDS: The Making of a Chronic Disease,* edited by Elizabeth Fee and Daniel M. Fox. Berkeley: Univ. of California Press.

Turner, Charles F., et al., eds. 1989. *AIDS: Sexual Behavior and Intravenous Drug Use.* Washington, D.C.: National Academy Press.

Turshen, Meredeth. 1991a. "Gender and Health in Africa." In *Women and Health in Africa,* edited by Meredeth Turshen. Trenton, N.J.: Africa World Press.

Turshen, Meredeth, ed. 1991b. *Women and Health in Africa.* Trenton, N.J.: Africa World Press.

Ulack, Richard, and William F. Skinner, eds. 1991. *AIDS and the Social Sciences.* Lexington: Univ. Press of Kentucky.

Ulin, Priscilla R. 1992. African Women and AIDS: Negotiating Behavioral Change. *Social Science and Medicine:* 34 (1):63–73.

UNICEF. 1993. "Street Youth and AIDS." Infold in *AIDS & Society* (January/February).

United Nations Development Programme (UNDP). 1991. "The HIV Epidemic as a Development Issue." Infold in *AIDS & Society* (October/November).

United Nations Development Programme (UNDP). 1992. "Young Women: Silence, Suceptibility, and the HIV Epidemic." Infold in *AIDS & Society* (October/November).

United States Catholic Conference. 1987. *The Many Faces of AIDS: A Gospel Response.* A Statement of the Administrative Board. November. Washington, D.C.: The Conference.

United States Department of State. 1992. *The Global AIDS Disaster: Implications for the 1990s.* Publication No. 9955. Washington, D.C.: The Department.

Vaid, Urvashi. 1987. "Prisons." In *AIDS and the Law,* edited by Harlon L. Dalton et al. New Haven, Conn.: Yale Univ. Press.

Valleroy, Linda A. 1988. "AIDS Case Reporting and HIV Surveillance in Developing Countries." In *AIDS 1988,* edited by Ruth Kulstad. Washington, D.C.: American Association for the Advanement of Science.

van de Walle, Etienne. 1990. "The Social Impact of AIDS in Sub-Saharan Africa." *Milbank Quarterly* 68 (Supplement 1):10–32.

Vladeck, Bruce. 1989. "The Economics of a Caring Approach." In *Public and Professional Attitudes toward AIDS Patients*, edited by David E. Rogers and Eli Ginzburg. Boulder, Colo.: Westview Press.

Wachtler, Robert M. 1991. *The Fragile Coalition: Scientists, Activists, and AIDS.* New York: St. Martin's Press.

Waite, Gloria. 1988. "The Politics of Disease." In *AIDS in Africa*, edited by Norman N. Miller and Richard C. Rockwell. Lewiston, Me.: Edwin Mellen Press.

Walters, LeRoy. 1988. Ethical Issues in the Prevention and Treatment of HIV Infection and AIDS. *Science* 239 (February 5):597–603.

Way, Peter, and Karen Stanecki. 1991. "The Demographic Impact of AIDS in Sub-Saharan Africa." Infold in *AIDS & Society* (April/May).

Weeramunda, Joe. 1990. Prostitution and AIDS in Sri Lanka. *AIDS & Society* (April):5–6.

Weisfeld, Victoria D., ed. 1991. *AIDS Health Services at the Crossroads: Lessons for Community Care.* Princeton, N.J.: Robert Wood Johnson Foundation.

Wermuth, Laurie, et al. 1992. "Women Don't Wear Condoms: AIDS Risk among Sexual Partners of IV Drug Users." In *The Social Context of AIDS*, edited by Joan Huber and Beth E. Schneider. Beverly Hills, Calif.: Sage Publications.

Wilson, Ronald W. 1988. "Measuring Risk Behaviors in Population-based Surveys." In *AIDS 1988*, edited by Ruth Kalstad. Washington, D.C.: American Association for the Advancement of Science.

World Health Organization, Global Programme on AIDS. *Report.* An annual publication.

Worth, Dooley. 1990. "Minority Women and AIDS: Culture, Race, and Gender." In *Culture and AIDS*, edited by Douglas A. Feldman. New York: Praeger.

Xavier, Ramnik J. 1992. "AIDS and Tuberculosis: A Dangerous Synergy." In *AIDS in the World*, edited by Jonathan Mann et al., 148-163. Cambridge, Mass.: Harvard Univ. Press.

Yeager, Rodger. 1988. "Historical and Ecological Ramifications for AIDS in Eastern and Central Africa." In *AIDS in Africa*, edited by Norman N. Miller and Richard C. Rockwell. Lewiston, Me.:

Edwin Mellen Press.

Yemane-Berhan, Tebebe. 1988. "HIV Infection in Developing Countries: Emerging Clinical Picture in Africa." In *The Global Impact of AIDS*, edited by Alan F. Fleming et al. New York: Alan R. Niss.

Zacarías, Fernando. 1989. "AIDS in Latin America." *AIDS & Society* (October):4, 24.

Zalduondo, Barbara O. de, et al. 1990. "AIDS in Africa: Diversity in the Global Pandemic." In *Living with AIDS*, edited by Stephen R. Graubard. Cambridge, Mass.: MIT Press.

Zenilman, Jonathan, et al. 1992. Effect of HIV Posttest Counseling on STD Incidence. *Journal of the American Medical Association* 267 (February 12):843–849.

Zinberg, Norman E. 1990. "Social Policy: AIDS and Intravenous Drug Use." In *Living with AIDS*, edited by Stephen R. Graubard. Cambridge, Massachusetts: MIT Press.

Name Index

Subject Index

Acquired Immunodeficiency Syndrome. *See* AIDS

ACT-UP (AIDS Coalition to Unleash Power), 93

Adolescents, 64, 189–90, 198–9

Africa: AIDS cases in, 11; blood transfusions in, 39; condoms associated with contraception in, 195; heterosexual transmission of HIV in, 25–27; HIV infections in, 11; military in, 34–35; orphans resulting from AIDS in, 48

African-Americans. *See* Blacks

African society: adultery in, 29–30; age gap between spouses in, 26; as an "alternative civilization," 27, 30–31; ancestry and descent in, 28; attitudes toward sex in, 28, 31; circumcision in, 27; chastity and sexual abstinence in, 28; Christian morality in, 30; commercial sex workers in, 29, 31; divorce in, 31; elites in, 44–45; health care expenses in, 50; higher education in, 44; homosexuality in, 25; hospital beds in, 48–49; polygyny in, 28; sexual relations in, 25–31, 28–29; transactional sex in, 28–29

Age distribution of AIDS cases, 63

Agriculture, 44

AIDS: African origin theory of, 32, 103–5; cases in the U.S., 55; cases worldwide, 6; comparisons with other diseases, 127–30; comparison with other epidemics, 130–32; concept derived from the West, 205; definition of, 5; as example of human vulnerability to the microbial world, 17–18; as harbinger of future epidemics, 16–18; incubation period of, 9 n.5; as international health problem, 116,119; pathology of, 127–30; problems in statistics of, 4–6; prospects for vaccine or cure for, 173–176; symptoms of

About the Author

YOLE G. SILLS is a sociologist and researcher and was Director of Interdisciplinary Studies at Ramapo College of New Jersey. A student of social change, she has produced several public television programs on AIDS and has directed numerous research projects on the role of medicine in American society.